Till I Grow

One woman's
triumphant
battle over
cancer,
her children
stood strong!

R. McAuley

outskirtspress

DENVER, COLORADO

You've held my hand,
walking me through unchartered territory of survival,
and used it for your glory.
You've blessed me beyond measure,
the author and finisher of my faith,
thank you Lord.

Acknowledgements

To my three amazing children, you've shown forth an abundance of courage, filled with grace, standing by mama through thick and thin. I'm overwhelmed with love for you. Through sickness, and health you were there. To all of the survivors, no matter how you've come to be, you were my light in a dim place. Just knowing of your existence, caused me to hold high my own banner of survival! My heart fills to overflowing, with thoughts of Tyler Rogers and Brenda Fox, who brought the sun shining back into my life, reminding me of the wonders of God. To every stranger who stepped on the scene (which felt like a million at times) and did their best in showing support, I thank you from the bottom of my heart. Thank you Terri Abstein my publishing consultant, at outskirts press.

You've been a pleasure to work with, always thorough during every aspect of my publishing experience. Also, many thanks to my outskirts press marketing team. I'd like to show forth my gratitude, in acknowledging the following companies, for allowing me to share their wisdom, and good intention. To Robert Harrison of get healthy again (and candida yeast), thank you for your quick responses, to e-mails and for all of your rich information. From my experience, your products really do work!

Elyse Bender-Segall, I'm grateful to you for granting me an opportunity of mentioning Xylitol, the natural sweetener. Thank you Goop, for adding a spice of life to my kitchen, with your wholesome recipes and plethora of tips to idyllic travel destinations. An abundance of gratitude, to owners of health recipes.com, for all of your wonderful healthy tips, and informative articles. To George M. for making the world a healthier place, with Whfoods. Karen Masterson, founder of Aloe Life thanks a million, for raising my awareness for such a time as this.

Thank you Reesa Lake of Black Girl Long Hair, for your continual encouragement, through articles of wearing natural tresses with confidence. Faeries dance, for keeping our skin covered with your wonderful organic fashion wear. Thank you Anthony Morrocco and staff of Morrocco Method, for leaving the customer well informed with your limitless expertise, and making them feel like their the only one, special. Many thanks to Karen from Green Peoples' site, I found yours to be most interesting, thank you again! Thank you Health Minute Vitamin Creek, for The Energy Neutralizer safety device, Lord knows we need! Mike from alkaline foods.net, I appreciate you! In saving the very best for last, I'd like to thank Master Prophet Bishop E. Bernard Jordan of Zoe Ministries, who has become my mentor, over the course of recent years. Thank you for your prophetic guidance, in helping me to find, what The Lord had already ordained for my life. Many thanks to your wife Pastor/Prophettess Debra Jordan, and the company of prophets, continued blessings to you all!

Table of Contents

Introduction

"NOTHING BEATS A failure but a try."

Moms' inspiring words of long ago, still ring true in the present, and will always give new meaning, new hope. Understanding one's destiny at first, can be somewhat complex, because you really don't know what's up ahead. However, a continual move forward, will eventually create a revelation. An awakening of that part of the mind, that had fallen asleep turning a deaf ear toward what it is that's bound to find you. But only if it's welcomed, long enough to allow the process of change to happen.

Facing an unexpected event can leave one feeling, defeated and hopeless. But once the realization of a clearer path presents itself, the feeling of 'it's too good to be true' arises. Why does it take an eye opener for some, to believe? Believing in miracles, signs and wonders of God, is a miracle in and of itself. Because some of us, maybe out of misunderstanding, have never had to walk in someone else's shoes, who had no other choice. Every single chapter of Till I Grow, was created through many real life circumstances. Every last one of them weren't overcome on the strength of myself, but of hanging in, and expecting my Lord to move on my behalf. It took a level of trust, and getting through tough times isn't fun, although it can bring about all that one needs in reaching their goals. And besides that, a true child of the Most High has a giant living on the inside, so why or how, could a true survivor give up? Persevering with unwavering determination, and a made up mind gets you to a place of awesomeness. Whenever an opportunity of change arrives, either we take it in and accept, or run as if our lives depended on it! On the other hand, when steps in the right direction are taken, that's when the sun will shine over the situation. No matter what the cost, we so deserve the best that life has to offer, why not take it? God is good, because He'll still be there waiting with open arms, meeting us when we need Him most, once we give everything to Him. His timing is not as ours, but He'll greet us wherever we are in our lives, Isn't that beautiful?! At your start and finished line, the good Lord is there. I've learned to let go, and if I should stumble, He'll catch me in His arms because He truly cares. Even if we don't love ourselves as we should, and are involved with the business and cares of this world, God is always there listening, waiting patiently, yearning to hear a word from our mouths to Him—anything. If nothing is said… still He waits. Oh

my God! That's what you call unconditional, depend-
able, infallible, and all else that would describe my
Father. Until we meet again, live life with boldness,
through your faith!

Scattered Seeds

A FOUL STENCH filled the air, as I crouched down on the floor clutching my belly. Mom in one corner, her date in the other. My older sister Tanya stood near the elevator doors, glaring down at me. Sharp words were exchanged, between mom and her boyfriend, as to why she took a fist to my stomach. A mere fight between two siblings, certainly didn't call for it, and Mom's argument began to escalate.

Meanwhile I caught my breath, desperately anticipating the opening of the elevator doors. Just as soon as they squealed open, I charged through the lobby echoing loud screams! At that point, we were outside as mom was fast approaching, taking great strides chasing me around a parked car. She yelled out to my sister to intercept, but there was no stopping me!

As I blazed past Tanya, mom's boyfriend quickly scooped me up! Shielding my tiny frame, to repel the next blow. After realizing there was no safety in his arms, I squirmed away dashing out into the street!

Seconds later, a heated beam warmed my face, just inches from impact. A police car had stopped short, directly in front of me and out stepped two officers, that escorted us to the police station.

During the ride all I could do is gaze out of the window, looking up at the street lights and beyond, into the darkened blue sky. Because it felt as though a black cloud were looming over us. My mind drifted past thoughts of playing with my dolls, and reading my favorite books, to what was going to happen to mom… us as a family?

The officers had promised Tanya and I, a couple of candy bars in attempts of cheering us up. I didn't fancy a treat, all I wanted was for my mother to re-surface, and for the stranger posing as her, to set her free. She became aggressive at times, for no particular reason at all and just wasn't herself, I knew something had changed about her. The short ride to the police station had become unbearable.

We were all stuffed in the backseat, and I couldn't wait to exit. Every so often I'd peer over at my mother, to see her grim expression staring back at me, without a flinch nor blink of an eye. The exact look she wore just before I made a run for it, out of the elevator. My attention regressed upward, toward the endless drea-ry sky. As soon as the car parked I hopped out, and one of the policemen, took Tanya and I by the hand leading us into the precinct. The second officer held mom's arm as they entered the office.

She sat at a desk in one room, while being questioned about what had taken place. Sister and I were in an office adjacent to where mom had been. Not long after, the officers congregated in one room, which left Tanya and I unattended. My mother walked out into the hallway, gesturing for us to follow her out of the precinct. Tanya quickly reached for mom's hand, and I followed her, but… stooped down to tie my sneakers. Then I untied them, then tied them again, my stalling continued long enough, for the policemen to complete their meeting or whatever they'd been doing. Mom gave me a striking look, when a couple of officers encamped around us, then took mom back into the office. That's when I asked the officer for a candy bar, and was determined not to leave with my mother. That'd also be the instance, of my survival torch being ignited, who knew? Things began to get interesting around that time, more than words can say. I had, had enough and a made up mind at six years old, on not returning to that apartment. Before morning, Tanya and I were taken to a hospital to await placement in a foster home. We lived there for one month on the pediatric unit.

Just before we were moved to our new home, mom visited us. I remember her walking in, with a clean shaven head and wearing a delightful smile. Out of distrust, I hid behind a food cart peaking through a small opening, just enough to assess the distance between us. Flashbacks ran through my mind, from the last we saw of each other, and how I was being hunted down like a runaway prisoner! I was not about to recap that event. That night was still fresh on my mind, and forgiving her would come years later. How to forgive became my dilemma, I didn't know how.

Besides God, she would be the only one to help me along with that. And for a long while, we weren't given the opportunity, to spend enough time for explanations. Tanya enjoyed the visit with mom, as they sat in the children's play room. I continued my stance, refraining from joining them, and thought to myself, as to why mom's hair was gone? Before all hell broke lose in our lives, she'd never mentioned going through chemo therapy. I chalked it up as her just expressing herself, what did I know?

I figured, she'd coin a new fashion statement, and given my age, it was totally over my head. One thing about my mother though, she had been way before her time, when it came to dressing and home décor. She was a fashion connoisseur in her own right! Her exquisite eye for the finer things in life, was out of this world! She could dress her tail off! A definite trait that she passed down to her children. And our apartment, had all the makings of a fierce interior decorator.

You'd think you were entering a celebrities house. A huge camel brown leather sofa, with an ottoman filled the living room. The walls were adorned with exotic artsy portraits. And mom added her elegant touch to our bedrooms, creating a spacious doll house. I loved it, and missed being at home. She truly had been a talented woman, but had no idea. So much time had flew by, before we'd see mom again, then I wished I hadn't been so stubborn, refusing her visit. Unfortunately, she had lost control of where her two daughters were going to live. I certainly wouldn't had been happy during a short visit, knowing that once the social worker said it was over, that's it. Mom would have to leave, we had to stay. So… for the time being I held a grudge toward her. We had no choice but to remain in that hospital, and our lives as we knew it, wouldn't ever be the same. The ultimate change in seasons had begun, and I believe we were all primed for that turning point, in which we were facing. Something truly had to give, there's no way on earth of how that situation could've continued on. It had arrived in a way, totally unforeseen from a six and eight year old. Clinging to hopes that mom would bounce back, after her and dad's divorce, had been my expectations back then. It wasn't completely understood by Tanya and I, we just stopped seeing dad come around. Visits from him lessoned as time rolled onward. My mother was truly a genuine delightful person though, until they split. It seemed as if all of her personality, and wit diminished while dealing with heart break. As time progressed, she mentioned how she had been diagnosed with cervical cancer, although I wouldn't quite get that part until I approached womanhood. And it made perfect sense, because she needed major help from pops, but he had moved on. A few months prior to the night of the chase, mom had promised to take Tanya and I on a trip. Instantly we had began discussing it on nights before going to bed, day in and day out, we were so excited, that we had worked ourselves into a frenzy! We discussed it during play time, over meals, going and returning from school. Finally, the day had arrived for our unknown suspenseful journey, and mom dressed us in beautiful attire. She had worked her artistry, in taming down our huge bushy 70's styled afros, and decorated our thick ponytails with sprinkles of colorful barrettes. Not long after boarding a train from Far Rockaway Queens NY, we made our way to Jamaica Queens our home town. While crossing the street I can remember mom holding our hands, guiding us as usual. She would always have so much to say. We'd walk, and talk, about any old thing we'd like. It became a ritual, and mom had the knack for making our travels interesting, as time sped by. On occasion Tanya and I would complain, that our feet hurt, or we're tired and mom would remind us of how, if we talked a little, we'd reach our destination sooner, boy was she right! But on that particular day, time seemed to drag by as if at a standstill. Mom remained silent, and I began to ask her questions, while attempting to pinpoint her mood in keeping the momentum going.

Every answer grew more intense, as we drew closer to the huge building that was in our view. I could tell that her usual self, had taken a backseat, and wanted to know why the change all of a sudden? Tanya and I both continued down the bustling city street. I thought to myself, "this must be the trip, our fun place!" As we stood hesitantly, in front of the building that towered over us, there were children with adults, entering and exiting. Some wore smiles, others were crying, altogether that had left me bewildered. Why would anyone be crying, if this place was such a fun dwelling for the children? Mom grew hesitant before chaperoning us inside, as if we were possibly at the wrong location. We followed her into an elevator, and when the doors reopened we stood in a long corridor. From the sounds of telephones ringing, and listening to the conversations on the other sides of the office doors, I began to realize our fun trip was something else. I could tell by the look on mom's face, that she was terribly unhappy, but why? What was mom thinking?

She turned to push a button on the wall for the elevator, and told us to wait there, someone would come for us. Right away I grabbed her hand, and Tanya followed suit. Once that elevator door opened, we all climbed on. Mom just looked at us, then went on to explain of how our trip had been cancelled, and she kept apologizing. After a while we didn't care about a trip, we wanted to go home with mom! She wasn't getting rid of us that fast honey! We all marched right back down to the train station, and went on with our mother. She had laid it all out, once I became an adult. During one of my many visits back home, she explained that mysterious trip. Turns out, mom was willingly going to have Tanya and I placed in foster care, through the children's services in that building. I wonder though, what had been going through her mind at that juncture, to the point of wanting to give us up? What did she feel as a mother? As she jogged my memory of that day, I realized mom had been crying out for help, but couldn't bring herself to go through with it. I remember telling her I wished she would've. Our lives may possibly have been more promising had she received assistance. We would've been able to return home sooner, without all of the years of getting stuck in the system. She had the burden of worrying about her health, and caring for us simultaneously.

Mom honestly could've kept afloat without extra responsibility. But like the good mother she was, she tried to hang in and complete what she set out to do... raise her two daughters as best she could. Before the onset of her battle with cancer, mom always found time to spend with Tanya and I. The best times had been when she'd read books to, and with us.

Causing her stories to come alive, with various facial expressions, and gestures. She had a magnetic way about her that drew you in, but in a short span of time... it had vanished. Couldn't help but wonder, would the old mom ever return? Eventually yes... she did, but with a scar across her heart that had cut so deeply, that it ate away at her more rapidly then her having cancer.

For comfort, I'd lean to my imagination to take me anywhere I'd like to be, while reading a book, using that forum as an escape. There were numerous instances when delving into a great read was associated with my mother. That's really all that had been available to grasp hold to after entering foster care. My way in some type of psychological form, of being near my mom. Reading a book, put me in touch with the familiarities of her.

And what she had planted in Tanya and myself, had become deeply rooted. She taught us of how a book, especially one with interesting photos, could take us anywhere, traveling for hours on end. I masked reading , with dealing with heavy issues. As the saying goes, a picture has a thousand words, I could've probably come up with 1,010!

If I saw a portrait or a beautiful antique painting, of say… for instance, a location in Italy, or anyplace other than where I had been, that's where my imagination lured me. To far away travels, beautiful homes, country sides, warm natives, and aromas of fresh baked goodies. My siblings there actually liked me, and our parents were truly in love and wanted a family. I knew mom wanted us, but dad on the other hand… well I'll just say he was a rolling stone, for real.

I can remember the still moments I'd spend, writing poems, theatrical plays, or anything that revived my spirit. While the other children were running about outside playing freeze tag or stickball, I was in my own world. There were times when mom and dad would be at work, and my great grand mother would baby sit, she'd always complain because of my excessiveness with books, Imagine that? I can't get enough of reminding my children, of how knowledge is power, and wouldn't dare discourage their enlightenment. But... I used to hear it all too often, sometimes she'd make me go outside to play, then I'd get bored and retract to my little reading workshop. Play time always ended with dramatics anyway, which may be the norm because children will be children. Someone had either gotten hurt running for the ball, or didn't like taking orders from my older sister Tanya. She forever in a day had to be the head boss in charge, so I kind of shied away from interacting on a regular. When the annual spelling bee rolled around, I'd study for days. Never won, but would always come in second or third, and that was just as good as winning. It never deterred me though, because I felt like a winner and welcomed the competition, it made things all the more exciting! And getting the jitters on stage, as everyone watched and listened, had my adrenaline racing, I loved it!

I didn't care if I lost, and just found a spelling bee to be fun. Whenever pondering a book of interest, I some how knew from the flow of the author, of whatever story I had chosen for that particular journey, if it would grab me. No doubt about it, I had to be clutching my hat and my dolls, holding on tight for my next ride! A ride of excitement, fairy tales, mystery, and all the trimmings of a great adventure! I literally had to be in flight with my read.

Once there, I'd visualize what my heart desired, the world was mines! Anything was possible, is what my mom would chant, whenever she'd be faced with a challenge. And so… it just stuck with me throughout. One thing about mom though, no matter what was going on she would set aside time to go over homework, and drill in our heads of how to pronounce difficult verbiage. The best of all… is when she'd ask us questions to see if we fully understood what was rehearsed.

If for any reason she felt we didn't grasp the story, we'd go over it some more. Those early memories of times spent with my mother, are worth more then all the money in the world, priceless! When I became of age and settled into my own skin, reading almost became a thing of the past though. Familiarizing myself, with dividing a paycheck was it! Once those adult years snuck up on me, I needed to do an inventory of what tickled my fancy.

Sure I love my children, and once dedicated myself to my ex-husband, but who was going to put a twinkle in my eye? Who's really up to the task, of treating me the way I honestly deserve? Me honey! I found numero-uno to be the answer to my own query.

So what I do now, at this stage of my life, are things that increase my contentment.

From time to time I curl up with a good novel, in between my busy schedule. And no more dreaming, I can really travel to far away places. Physically there vacationing and not escaping, that's what adulthood gave me, freedom! Well part of vacationing is a form of escape, from that which is mundane, the status quo of responsibilities... the norm. Finally I can live, I'm free... not allowing anyone to stifle my aspirations! It seemed forever and a day, where I could actually say that. I'm telling you, after you have walked these pages with me, you'll get the full picture of why I'm filled to capacity, and over flowing with joy! And I hope you will be ready to reach new heights in your life as well. Like a trumpet, it's high time of sounding the alarm of survival! All of the unforeseen experiences in my younger years, has me on a mission of no return! Thankfully the past is gone, however... I use it as a tool in tightening up the loose ends in the here and now. When I was a little girl, I had no choice but to use my imagination, in guiding me through heartbreak, or for anything that caused concern or worry. And to be so young, I worried just as much as I do now! And about serious big stuff that I shouldn't have had on my mind, at five and six years of age. I was an old soul, that's what my great grandmother Mama, would call me. Maybe it came from the many talks I'd have with my mom, about anything, which matured me beyond my years. I had become her companion, and she'd discuss very interesting things, and would ask me questions. Having that type of relationship, readied me for my adult life.

Also by witnessing, how dedicated she had been to my dad, was a good example, of how a woman should treat a man. By watching my grand/great grandparents, portrayed how a man should honor a woman. My grandparents had the utmost respect for one another. And if I didn't learn anything else, dad taught me how to not throw my pearls before swine, so I thank you for that dad. Not to say I've never fallen for the okeydoke, because I have, and more than once.

With mom our minute years together lasted long enough, as she taught me what I needed to know in the nick of time, before our separation... how to be a survivor. It prepared me for the world, although I had been so young, yet in still I got it. For something that had began in such a sublime manner, almost ended in tragedy though, with me on the short end of the stick. Honestly, I could've lost my life on many different occasions, but it was not meant to pan out that way, thanks to my faith which had begun early on. I mean... I needed someone, something to grasp hold to, that wouldn't fail me or cause deep rooted pain. For once or maybe twice, or as many times as necessary, I can live a meaningful life! In such a way, that it feels surreal and it is. I'm on my own at this point of my life, in full control of IT but wouldn't have it any other way. And as a child, growing up in New York City was extremely difficult. You'd better be skilled and well crafted, to survive the concrete jungle!

Wouldn't it be great if there were a map offering ways in which to maneuver, in avoiding pitfalls, crazy twists and turns? Some genius really needs to invent such a device, am I right? What's your take on it? It may sound far fetched, but the possibilities are endless, especially with vast expansion in technology. Why not create something that can audibly, redirect your path? Beware, of danger up ahead! Or, he's a dog, kick him to the curb!

I would so welcome that as I'm certain you would as well. I believe in due time what I've just described, will be looked at as acceptable in the near future. It would save one from a world of trouble, and who knows what else. Unfortunately, I had my bouts with the system, as far as foster care was concerned, and I was too young to look out for any red flags. Although I'm sure they were there, flailing wildly in my face, but back then I didn't get it. And mother had been diagnosed, with cervical cancer prior to my sister and I, having to be placed in foster care. When I became older she explained to me her big plans of how she'd been looking forward, to growing old with my dad. Once my parents divorced, it left the brunt of raising my eldest sister Tanya, and I to fall on moms' shoulders. This is where she became overwhelmed, and begin releasing her stress, onto me. The result of that changed everything. Who knew my sister and I wouldn't return to mom, until after eight years. I couldn't bear being away from my children for eight days, and when mom opened up, and rehashed, I felt her pain. Although it would be years until that moment of release, nevertheless it came, I understood. My adulthood cleared the confusion, that had gone through my mind as a child, and naturally so. Mom encountered much heartache, which unfortunately became part of her destiny.

I do believe that her way of life, could have been much better. She needed someone to be cheering her on, as far as her parents were concerned. At least that's what I gathered, from the long talks we'd have over the years, concerning her relationship with her parents. She didn't have the grounded support, that she so desperately searched for. The only real substance available to her, was total dysfunction that caused her to be estranged from certain individuals, that she put all her trust in. It really does take a village, everyone pulling together being an anchor for the one who's fallen… keeping them afloat. By my mother losing ground, it created a domino effect that stops HERE! I'm not sure exactly what sent her over the edge. Could it have been her own cancer diagnosis, the divorce, or both? She had strategically distanced herself, and with good reason. To be totally honest, my mom was a mysterious being, at least to me. I'm not sure if it's because of our short time spent, or if it's because she really was a force to be reckoned with. I began to understand her rhyme of reason, as did my siblings Tanya, Tiffany, and Jahvon. Of course a child after a while, gets what drives the one who birthed them into the world. It took some time, and what I'd remember as a teen, to see clearly through the stained glass of what mom was made of. One thing is certain, I remember her as classy, pure at heart, and as wholesome as could be. I'll always reminisce of my mother this way. It's a known fact, that the first six years of a child's life are vital in receiving what they need, in all aspects of development.

I believe it to be true, because I did get to see who Sandra M. Warford, was, from my birth until I was six years old. The real Sandra, before we were separated. Mom attempted to hold it together for us, and I can still hear her strong, baritone voice quoting, "nothing beats a failure, but a try." Out of all of her numerous quotes, that one stuck with me and has become the anthem that pulled me through. Through the years spent in foster care, and later on a dreadful breast cancer diagnosis.

Our lives were sent on a roller coaster, that literally tore us apart. I had been abused, at the hands of my mother, but it didn't come over night, I witnessed her frustrations, and saw her fighting with every reserve to try and hang in there. Her anger and pain had to be released some how, unfortunately I was on the receiving end. But she… in my eyes at six years old, was mom and I absolutely adored her… still. We had a tight bond, never to be severed or so, I perceived in my juvenile psyche.

I could sense that she'd been trying to make up for lost time, in the way she vibed with my eldest daughter, after her birth. That's what made it easy for me to forgive, because I saw her morph into the mother, that she couldn't be with me. And I saw the highs and lows of mom, so I knew she was on the verge of something, when the abuse began. It was totally out of her character. She had to deal with divorce, and adjusting to a single parent life style.

Her cancer diagnosis had arrived a few years later, along with alienating herself from her family. She thought it was best to try and survive on her own, and I always gave her credit for that. I knew first hand what it felt like to deal with rejection, when sending out an S.O.S. to no avail. And to have kept it moving, shows great courage, with anyone who's facing a hardship. With the proper guidance, I'm sure the portrait of my mom's story, would've been read with a lighter back drop.

I believe in changed destiny, and If you want something badly enough, until the point you can breathe, feel, and taste it… until it protrudes through your pores, yes it's Possible! Have you ever been there, do you get where I'm coming from? You won't and can't afford, for anything nor anyone to distract your focus.

But only if your at the place, where you believe in yourself, and you kick defeat out of the way.

Yes you can change your destiny, especially when there's someone on your team, that makes their presence be known, and felt. It can be one person and you, which makes up a pair, and your in! That one confidant, that's got your back when it's up against a wall. In mom's case she didn't have much of that, and just kind of gave up. Not totally, but she did leave room for more than what she'd expect.

And with her attempting effort, I will never forget her struggle, as she toiled at being a good mother, and she was in my eyes. Now I realize, just how important it is for me to add a twist, to how things unfold in my life. At each opportunity that presents it self, I shake up and shake off, the old generational cycles from my family. I will not at all, allow the same nightmares to rare their ugly heads, with how I raise my children. Sure we've had our ups and downs, however,

I always go that extra mile in pushing, squeezing a little more out of myself, until we get it together. Then again sometimes you have to do what's best, and safe for all involved. You just have to let go at times, if the other person is unwavering, causing an unbalanced flow. You have to move on, and wish them well… whom ever it is that you must separate from, if you want to be happy.

I've also learned the hard way of letting go too late, never the less I've learned. No one comes to mind that I know, who'd be all smiles if faced with an unwanted, unexpected change. An upheaval if you will. Not long after being placed into foster care, I had an emergency surgical procedure, and to make matters worst, mom wasn't allowed to be with me.

Internal bleeding had occurred, from a scuffle I had with a neighbor. I remember getting punched in the stomach, where I'd already had one blow too many, and that one had broken the camels back. I did not want to get the other child in trouble, out of fear of what my foster parents would do to me. I quickly conjured up a story, assuming they would punish me as usual.

Nice try, but they didn't buy it. If it had not been for me having to be rushed to the emergency room, I'm sure they would've been after me for fighting. All of those numerous occasions of riding the bus and train with mom, had paid off as she taught Tanya and I, how to pay attention to street signs, and remember land marks. It was fun, learning how to navigate my way around Queens New York. And thankfully that's where our foster home was, so we were already in the know, on how to maneuver through Queens.

Had it had been a Bronx or Manhattan foster care placement, I'm sure we would've gotten lost. None the less, traveling other parts of New York, would come at a much later time. Prior to having surgery I had run away, and was fed up with getting beaten, for everything I did, or didn't do. I stood on the lawn calling to my sister Tanya, and she poked her head out of the window, looking down at me. I said to her, "I'm leaving, and going to Mama's house." She lived about twenty minutes away from the foster home. Which was quite a distance for a six year old to walk alone. And at the time that was my safe place, where I knew grandma would set things straight, for sure. But Tanya answered, "I'm not going, you go!" And that's what I did, without realizing I had spiked a fever.

While walking, I heard my mother's voice, telling me to look both ways, before crossing those huge city streets. Pay attention to the people around you. And don't talk to strangers, that was the big one. So... I was maybe five blocks away from mama's house, and a man standing in his yard asked was I lost? I hit panic mode, retracting my steps, and quickly walked back to the drawing board, to devise my next escape. I really wanted out of that foster home, and had been missing my mother awfully bad. Unfortunately, for what happened next, I didn't need a new runaway plan at all. My sister greeted me outside in the yard, singing a tune, "your in trouble, your gonna get it!"

My foster mother's first reaction was to grab a belt, as I watched her angry expression, change into a horrified one.... one that I hadn't seen before! There was blood trickling down my legs, coming from my vaginal area, and she kept asking what happened? Finally I confessed to her, the fight I had earlier that day and began describing my excruciating abdominal pain.

She quickly washed me up, and changed my clothing. Shortly after, an ambulance screeched to a halt , and whirlwind me to the hospital. As this thought comes to mind, I believe she was worried that maybe the daily beatings, I'd received from her and her husband, is what caused the internal bleeding. I'm not sure, but as I think back it all makes sense to me now, she just seemed nicer than usual, behaving as a mother should when concerned for a child. No one explained to me what was happening. And as time progressed I learned that I had suffered extensive trauma to my stomach. Which caused me to wet the bed every day. To be totally honest, the bleeding could've come from any and all of the abuse. I can remember my foster parents, beating me in shifts. One day the mother would have a belt, come into my room abruptly pulling my blanket off of me, and as soon as her bulging eyes noticed the bed was wet, down came the belt. The next day her husband followed suit, and my sister would be nervously watching, with tears rolling down her face. I was taken from one abusive situation, to another. Never once did I report the beatings to my social worker.

I assumed wetting the bed was wrong, it was my fault and I deserved getting attacked every morning. I didn't know. Well… you can truly see how times have changed, because there's a major difference between a six year old from the seventies, as opposed to a six year old who has been born in more recent years. Oh yes… knowledge has definitely increased. Nowadays, children are swifter and will tell you where to go, and will take you there honey! I'm in no way glorifying that fact, because I believe in a child respecting their elders, sadly enough that's the way of the world. But not in my house, and I'm sure many decent parents will agree. That's the only way to put this thing in reverse, one house, one family, one person at a time, nothing is impossible. Fortunately there are much more services available, in which they can reach out to avoid having an experience like mines.

No one wants to see there loved one placed in foster care, but it happens. As long as the child is safe, and the biological family is receiving some type of counseling, eventually it will lessen the problem. Then core issues can be picked apart, and dealt with. Maybe not all at once, because most anything worth fighting or pushing for is a process.

But the healing will show up, especially if that's what all parties are looking for. Just before my surgery, those poor nurses and doctors had their hands filled! I was kicking, and screaming, and they some how were able to administer the anesthesia. My thoughts at the time were horrifying! I thought they were out to inflict more harm on me, and I didn't trust anyone.

But by the sound of mom's voice, or the aroma of her perfume, would've meant the world to me. I'm certain her being there would've settled me, because I hadn't seen her in so long. It was terrifying, not knowing what to expect! This had to be my punishment, for getting into a fight or so I thought. A silhouette of mom, crossed my mind as I called out to her, "mommy," before going under.

I missed her a great deal. I missed her braiding my hair, watching her cook up a meal in our kitchen, and going for our long walks. I used to love watching my mom as she'd play her oldies music, while doing her house cleaning on Saturdays. Every so often she'd peer over at Tanya and I, while holding the broom as a microphone, as she sang out loud. We'd crack up laughing, or join in because we knew the lyrics to all the songs. Lord knows she played them enough.

After all that had happened, Tanya and I were moved to another foster home. And following the surgery, my hospital stay lasted about two weeks. During that time for some odd reason, I couldn't walk so I sat in a wheelchair bored out of my mind. I missed riding my bike, my collection of books, freedom in general I guess. I hadn't gotten any visitors, and needed to see a familiar face. Outside of the nursing unit, was a pay phone... remember those?

So I called my great grandmother, maybe a day or two crept by, and both my grand and great grandmothers, Dorothy and Mama came walking through the nursing unit. It was like sunshine on a cumulus day! My social worker had to accompany them. And at six years old, I got the ball rolling by just making a phone call, and it was done! As long as I lay in that hospital bed, just waiting… no one would have come.

I've always been the type of person, to go for what I wanted, and not sit around looking to someone else to make it happen. My motto of today? Go get what's yours! By any decent , honest means necessary. It's astonishing as to how, a young child thinks. They have their very own way, of understanding their world and the people who reside in it. Doesn't always happen, but an adult needs to be held accountable, to steer them to a positive place. Do we live in a perfect world? Certainly not, but by me instilling healthy discipline into my children, I believe their lives will be less burdensome. God forbid , if they weren't paying attention, shame on them! At that time, mom hadn't been privy to my surgical procedure, and the severity that stemmed from the abuse as a whole. She lost something along the way…. it wasn't love, but it was something. Unfortunately many years went by, before family counseling came into play. Never the less, it enabled me to forgive. I'd probably be a different, kind of parent today if I didn't sever the grip of animosity back then. While writing this memoir, I took a brief hiatus to regroup, gain clarity and peace of mind. Although it broke my heart, I put my seventeen year old daughter, on a bus and sent her to live with her dad.

I once explained to my children, and made it crystal clear, that if there's someone in their lives, causing discomfort even if it's your own sibling, you must let go! Yes you love them, want to support, and simply be there for them. But… if your doing all of that, and they can't seem to get it together, give them space in allowing them to find their own way.

Just before writing my memoir, we were once again displaced, and I mean struggling, living in hotels, and staying with a relative. The year before last I had surgery, and was hospitalized for four days. Two days after I was discharged, my relative and I had a disagreement. They put my three children, and myself out on the street at one in the morning.

I had stitches in my stomach, and other highly sensitive areas. Driving, definitely was out of the question, but given the circumstances, there was no choice. We ended up going to the emergency room, because I was in so much pain. I was on the verge of giving up, but all I could think about were my three children, and pray that my God would help us, and soon!

I gave my relative a call, asked if we could come back, and they said yes, I was so grateful! At every opportunity , I was on the internet in search of an apartment. A year prior, I had applied at different apartment complexes. The waiting lists were too long. Three weeks after surgery, my children and I, took a long drive to visit another relative.

During that time, I completed an application for an apartment. We were staying at a hotel, for the visit. Two weeks after returning to my other relatives house, I was approved for the apartment, Hallelujah! My prayer was to have a place, to call home before Thanksgiving and Christmas, and now we had it again. It took me five years, to have the courage, to send my first baby girl, to stay with her dad.

In spite of cancer treatment, homelessness, holding down a job, and nurturing three children on my own, my eldest child's behavior became unbearable. I remember telling her "you were there you saw it all, are you so serious?" As a teen I was no angel, but come on now. Enough was enough, I had to maintain stability for my two younger children.

She's reached the borderline of being a young woman, yet is still having to follow my rules at home. It wasn't seventeen minutes, nor seventeen hours. I raised her for seventeen YEARS, now it was papa's turn. I sometimes wonder, did I teach her enough? Was she paying attention? Did I show her enough love? In spite of all that's happened, our communication has greatly improved, and I do miss her, but let me tell you… I have no regrets.

I also made it my business, to reassure her that if she needed me, she knew where I'd be. But… I have no intentions in coddling her, I believe she's had enough of that. Now she must experience some things on her own, which in my opinion is very healthy for her, at this juncture. Survival had been a way of life, for me all through out. And with the scattering about, from foster home, to foster home, time didn't allow forming lasting relationships. Until moving to the third one. That particular placement, birthed a plethora of great memories, and some weird ones also. My third foster mother is now in her eighties. After thirty years, we continue keeping in touch. She was a mother to me , and still to this day. She loves telling stories, of how I was as a little girl. You should see the look, on my children's faces. "Get out, no way, mom not you, how?!" were their queries.

They find it difficult to fathom, that I've lived the same stages they've experienced thus far. Different span in time, thank heavens! Yes kiddos, mama has traveled up, and down that road before. I'm also thankful that my childhood era, didn't began in the Millennium. So much so, that I must... say it twice! I'm happy to be me, as an adult than to be a teen, right now, can you imagine?

Than again, who knows, how life would have turned out. Maybe my mother would've raised me, and remained that sweet gentle flower, full of love and inspiration. But the subtle easy going, mother of mines, became hardened of heart. Who could blame her? She didn't get a fair shake, at the dawn of her own life. It's doable, but difficult to mirror by example a way of living, that you were never exposed to.

Even the tiniest instances, when a person absorbs something positive into their lifestyle, will positively effect the next individual. No matter how small the gesture, they'll be enlightened some how. Eight long years go by, and I was knee deep in the foster care system. Although weekend visits home, were met with anticipation, living with strangers had become the norm.

But with age, my stance in the world had meaning. Especially after being placed, with a family that played a vital role, in helping me to exhale… at first. But… lo and behold, dysfunction! They had it too! As mentioned earlier, reading was my forte. And the stories took me to a place, of the unknown. I remember rushing through chores, and getting back to a book marked page, to continue my journey.

I found adventure in reading stories, that were filled with the like. Though, in the many learned words, and phrases, I'd never come across the word dysfunction. I had an idea, it had to be in the books. And I guess in the seventies, the most fitting word would had to have been, chaotic … Yes that'd be it! Unfortunately everyone's familiar, with some form of confusion, in their families. But knowing how to rid yourself of it, is key.

Whenever anything out of the ordinary occurred, I'd think to myself "no, I will do things different, when I get big." Many situations I witnessed back then, my children will not have to be subjected to. I've shown them documentaries, of how other children are barely making it, and thousands of their parents, may not even be alive. In most cases there isn't foster care available, for them. The only option may be, to survive the best way they can. By now we all know that, knowledge is power. This is what I reiterate, to my children. I made it clear, that they'll have choices, and I hope they choose smart ones. When the time arrived, for me to live back with my mother, I was convinced of a smooth transition.

Mom, Tanya and I, were on our way toward a positive thing now. Hitting all green lights, everything was good! And… with the talks, and prep of returning home, no one ever said, "Hey kid… don't forget to pack light!" It took a few months before realizing, that my heart was no longer at home. The abuse wasn't as bad, but prevalent.

The years spent visiting, didn't compare to the actual permanency of this new change. Not very much planning, went into moving my sister and I back home. Or so, that's how it seemed. It felt as if the social worker, was throwing us back into an uncertainty. Instead of writing, of how I survived breast cancer, and foster care, my book could be about, how overwhelmed the system is.

Resulting in thousands of children, falling through the cracks. I pray this memoir, encourages someone who may feel like letting go. Wait… hold on! Read my story friend, don't give up! On this journey, curiosity had my stomach in knots. With every ounce of my being, of my existence, I wanted to know just how it was all going to unfold? If I had given up to turn around, what would've transpired? What did I have prior? Nothing, but now I had hope, that pushed me forward.

With the much needed help, from the God I know. As the one and only, who is capable of sustaining me all of these years. The God that I personally believe in, and pray to was, and still is my mother and father. Shortly after returning home, I ran away. Eventually I was herded into a home for teens, and It happened so quickly. Tanya went to stay with a relative, and we didn't get to see one anther too often.

My social worker, had grown just as fed up with me, as I were with her. Although I had been Labeled a troubled teen, that was not my given name at birth, I never accepted it. As my age began to place limits, on where I was to reside in the system, the sadden truths of being scattered and lost in the shuffle, hit like an anvil! I was once again at a crossroads, yet unbeknownst to me the temporary group home, was a new starting point, and for real this time.

Because I had become exhausted, with out a clue of knowing what to expect! My survival skills, were fine tuned at that point. I prepared myself, for whatever come what may. There were times, when I had to fight to protect myself from the tough girls. It became, an every girl for herself type of circumstance. Until one day I began to fight back uncontrollably, and disrespecting the staff members,

I didn't care about anyone. No one gave a roosters'

crow where I'd end up, so why should I have? I mean, I would say the most hurtful things, just to piss the staff off. Knowing they couldn't lay a hand on me. Not realizing of how badly, I was playing myself into a corner, of permanent time out! My grades in school, had down spiraled. I hit rock bottom, and was tired of getting pushed around. Overall, I was an easy going person, that had been quickly darkening the threshold, of something totally different. My social worker, threatened to have me placed in a juvenile detention facility. Which would've faired, much more worst than where I had been living, there would be no comparison. I heard it all before, promises of sending me to a juvenile center, whatever, okay, sure, I dare you, was my attitude.

I paid it no attention, and was not the least bit concerned, talk about naïve? When the day came, for me to be moved to the juvenile center, boy was I shutten up! No longer bellowing out sarcastic remarks, toward the staff members. Most importantly, no longer covered under the age umbrella, or beside myself in thinking somebody owed me something. Sister girl had a rude awakening!

It took some time to understand that no one was obligated, to do anything for me. I had been displaced due to abuse, It was of the past, and the time had surfaced to fly, or crash and burn. And it didn't register with me, that a person may have to be court ordered, to a juvenile detention center. If I had known that, I probably would've carried on until they just booted me out!

I've never lived as a ruffian, or someone remotely close to that caliber, but had a little too much extra steam to blow off. Unfortunately in the wrong direction, toward folks that were only trying to help. And the staff were at their wits end, so something had to happen to bring old girl back. Nor did it ever cross my mind, that a judge set up a day visit which entails brunch, and a tour guide.

Picture a bug, on it's back scrambling, kicking out with wings flailing, it'll do whatever necessary to help itself! If not, it may be eaten alive, or stepped on. It's something how when your lying flat out, on your back, there's no place to go... but up! It's true, can't just lay there, you must get up! I was that bug going against the grain, as stubborn as I wanted to be, until reality slapped me to my senses, and quick!

Now as I was waiting on the front porch, to be chaperoned to the visit, I began scanning the neighborhood to see what I'd be missing. I saw people sleeping in boxes, homeless or on drugs, clearly in their own state of mind. But seemed at ease, with throwing in the towel, what's to miss? The ladies of the day, and night were out, and about.

Witnessing this, were the status quo. But.... if half the community, is just lying down unmotivated with life passing them by, it puts the next generation in limbo, and it did. Except for those individuals who refused to succumb to that. It was time to face the music, and the social worker stepped onto the side walk, motioning for me to follow.

We entered her car, and she begin reciting a speech of my down falls, and accomplishments. Just when I was beginning to enjoy her company, she informed me of mom's approval for the transition, I almost gagged! "Okay mom... are you so serious?!" Would've been my shocking reaction. Trust me the words didn't come close to anything respectable, I was done with her! Your having me... sent to where? I'm going to really, put on a show for the people now!

I had began thinking of a way, to behave negatively, in getting back at my mother. She knew that where I was, had been a little better, than living in a place filled with, Lord knows who or what. How did I get here? At that point, I had no choice as to where I was going, but the night mares I'd already encountered, helped me to put one foot in front of the other, and take a chance. The path behind, was strategically set before me. Forward march, no turning back! The visit took place, in the fall of nineteen eighty six, and what a gorgeous day! Gazing upon the naturally painted foliage, released anxiety. The two hour drive, through upstate New York felt awe inspiring! I never knew that part of New York even existed! Fear melted away as I sat near a window, opened to a crisp breeze, that danced across my face, and dried the tears of despair. If all else failed, I did enjoy the drive through the never before seen (at least by my eyes) picture-perfect idyllic New York, before meeting my doom. Each breath of fresh air had a soothing affect, that was desperately needed. While approaching young adulthood, there were frustrations and eagerness to just get on with it.

Absolving my mother for her short comings, was the focal point in moving forward. She too, had to go through a healing phase. I had to step aside, and allow the process. If I had it my way, mom and I would've been good friends, from high school or something. In the interim, that's exactly what we became. I would've told her, come on girl, stand under my umbrella.

I've got your back through your struggling time of need. She was a beautiful person inside out with loyalty, and good intentions. Although, not always receiving the same in return. One thing is certain, she made it easy for me to forgive. We must do it in keeping balance, with healing and growth. Forgiveness is a difficult lesson, that I had to become reacquainted with, in the recent years.

It's not easy, but we all have to face it… or not. It's a free will type of thing, no one is forced to let bygones, be bygones. On the other hand, much clarity comes with forgiveness, thus saving un-wasted energy. We were all dealt these hands for a purpose. You have yours, I have mines. What matters most is how to play, hang in there and win! Positive expectancy, is what orchestrates my life now. It's a daily immersion and I search high, and low expecting good things.

I'm not walking around all day with a wide smile, unfazed. But I try, and deal with anything, and everything with an open mind. It took hard work, on readjusting my own way of thinking. Which called for changing people, places, and things, literally. I had to, it became part of surviving. However... learning to let go of a situation that's out of my control, is still ongoing for me. That part of me, is what I wrestle with.

I can be stubborn at times, so there's still work to do in that area of my life amongst others, an ongoing process. My new home was in the distance, but didn't look like a juvenile facility. Groups of teens, were walking around as if on a college campus. There weren't any barb wired fences as I assumed, only a few buildings which had coed dorms, surrounded with rich green grass, and clusters of trees, sheer breath taking!

The total opposite of what I'd been used to in the city. The school had been in walking distance, in the structure of a country barn. An immense one though, with intimate classrooms, and I loved it! I wanted to thank my mother, for exercising her rights. She knew I'd have an opportunity, at a better life. I remember the look on my social workers' face which read, "I can't wait until this one's on her way." I know she wanted to say it, instead she gave me a look of disgust. I had a huge smile on my face, and wanted to take back everything I had said earlier. I hugged her as if she were mom, and pleaded with her not to mention a word.

I deserved the nerve wrecking suspense, of assuming I was going to a detention center. The social workers' way of repaying me, for giving her more grey hair. Because she knew all along, of where I'd be going. I was elated, moving on up and had found my niche!

At last... a happy place in time. Everyone seemed... different than what I'd portray in my mind, which had been the worst. They wore expressions of confidence, but had also been through some type of traumatic ordeal, which brought them to peace in the valley. That place of peace, became available for me. With an exception of the two girls, that were asked to tour me around.

From my angle, the residue of their past stood out on their faces. But... I wouldn't ever again, judge a book by it's cover. Despite their demeanor, both girls turned out to be, really helpful. They were patient, and kept reassuring me of how I was going to like living there. I had an opportunity in meeting almost everyone, teachers, counselors, and the principal.

Not a single stone, left unturned. New beginnings were under way, and at the top of my list, CHECK! It was time to exit the rollercoaster, no longer scattered here and there. This particular setting, turned out to be the leverage needed, in preparing for journeys ahead. It was all up to me now, and after my eye opening visit, I had been given two options.

Remain in the home from the hood, or move to where the opportunities were endless... honey I chose the latter! I must say, I had some fun crazy times at my new home. Two years after moving there, I remember sneaking out passed curfew with a roommate. We climbed out of our bedroom windows, to go meet our boyfriends for a rendezvous.

We were running down a dirt road, and clumsy me falls into a ditch springing my ankle. My roommate had to practically carry me back. To make matters worst, we had to ring the front door bell, to alert the night staff. At three in the morning, the facility director came from home, and drove me to the emergency room. It's hilarious now, but back then I was in all kinds of trouble that night.

They put up with me, for three and a half years. By having the pleasure of meeting, such understanding but firm patient staff, it has guided me through many adversities. Tough love helped to mold me, into the woman of today. Mom knew exactly what she was doing. Not only did she approve, she made requests and bugged the heck out of the agency, that were my partial legal guardians.

For me it signified that my mother did mean well, and always had the last word. She was mom! As time went on my grades picked up, and I developed a more amicable relationship with mom. She'd come visit me, and visa versa. We'd take lots of pictures, of the country scenery. I fell in love as promised, on the day of my tour and never wanted to leave. Finally home sweet home!

I was compelled to began my story, in the younger years, which primed me for the many battles that were to come. And to shed some light on how to try, and get through hardships. You may or may not fall, but incase you do, dust your self off and keep it moving! While growing up, I didn't always dwell in un-pleasantries. If my face wasn't glued to a book, I'd create fun, and excitement with my sister, and best friend Garrick "Spanky" Parker, from school. We met in the third grade, in Cambria Heights Queens NY, and are friends until this day. I have some of the best memories, one happened to be on July 13, 1977, the famous blackout in New York City.

Garry was 7, I was eight years old on that hot summer day, and all of the children were out riding bikes, just having honest fun. Of course it had caught everyone off guard, and without a care in the world, we all continued running around the neighborhood playing. And I remember the day, I had invited Garry over my house for a wedding, that took place in the living room, of my foster mothers' house, it was packed! My buddy and I literally danced, ate, and played all night into the morning hours.

One day on the way home from school, I fell and banged up both knees pretty badly. My best friend took me to his house, which had been on the way to mines, and his grandmother went to work on my knees. After she cleaned and bandaged my legs, Garry gave me a piggy back ride, all the way home.

I could hear him breathing heavy, by the time we reached my block.

He was exhausted, but carried me directly to my doorstep. He took care of me, as if I were special to him. And in turn he became my confidant, as I let him into my world. Filling him in on how I was a foster child. It didn't change anything though, we were still the best of friends, and he'd always know just what to say, in getting my mind off of missing my mother.

Garry was the salve to my inner wounds, little did he know. God truly blessed Tanya and I, we saw first hand of how family should be. His mother, and grandmother treated my sister and I as such. You could feel the love, when entering their home. That's what we needed, love and a family. After a number of years, I moved to the new group home, and we lost contact.

Three years ago our friendship, had been reunited on an internet social network. I was so happy, and in tears to find my ole friend of over 36 years! There's so many more events that took place in my blessed, highly favored life. However, I wanted to present my story to you in it's simplest form, as opposed to writing a Bible sized book. I wanted to give you a peek into my life, and as a total stranger.

Actually… you may know me, I'm that survivor whom you love dearly. Your sister, or mother? Perhaps a neighbor, or aunty… I could be your sister-cousin? Or the check-out clerk, who kindly greets you at the local market male/female. Unfortunately, cancer has no respecter of persons.

And at the time, I was not aware of men having breast cancer. I'd never heard of it, of course until sitting side by side, with a couple of male patients, during chemo treatments. One gentlemen was very young, maybe in his early twenties and was diagnosed with... yup you guessed it, breast cancer. But it makes sense, due to the fact that men have breast tissue, as do women.

Can you imagine a man though, getting a mammogram? There are various ways, in testing males for breast cancer. They can be tested by having an MRI or an ultra sound, which in my opinion is similar to a mammogram, but less intense. The Pet scan/PT Scan (Positron Emission Tomography) is another form of testing. With the PT Scan a liquid radiotracer is inserted intravenously. And what this does, is show whether or not, cancer has spread to vital organs. As with all medical treatment, and tests where radiation is used, there may or may not be side effects. Which are only two, the wanted, and unwanted. Hopefully the patient will receive no side effects.

Withering Diagnosis

IT'S BAFFLING, OF how one minute life's grand, all things love. I go to work, make time to spend with my children, the everyday routine, next thing you know... I had Breast cancer. In November of 2,005, I was diagnosed with a stage three breast cancer, which wasn't a good thing. Not only because of the initial diagnosis, but for the fact that the higher the level in stages, the more crucial receiving treatment became. I was thirty six, my children were, two, six, and ten years old.

And as a single mom after hearing the news, I began to wonder who will take care of us, if I wouldn't be able to? I hit panic mode, what were we going to do?! After working in the health care field, for over twenty years, I knew first hand of how to take care of someone receiving cancer treatment. But personally experiencing cancer, was an eye opener!

I had been a nurses aide, and would work at various nursing homes, and hospitals through a nursing agency. Following my diagnosis I'd get flash backs, of helping one of my patients who had cancer. Just the thought of all I had witnessed at work, almost sent me reeling over the edge! I go to lift the frail patient out of bed, sit them in their wheel chair, and help them to the bath room.

Or give a bed bath to try and comfort the individual. Dress them in warm clean pajamas, or spoon feed them a meal. Cancer had ravished through some patients so fiercely, that they were tube fed, or would have intravenous nourishments. This nightmare, played over, and over in my head. My primary care physician referred me to a surgical oncologist, that wanted to get in there, and cut the tumors out, immediately!

One was the size of a walnut, along side my left breast near the under arm area. The other measured the size of a lime, nestled over the top, of the same breast. I remember buying a bra, which I loved, and the very next day after wearing it, I had the worst excruciating burning sensation, and itching. That's when I noticed the two lumps.

It's as if they appeared over night! I sought a second opinion, which confirmed the initial diagnosis. As a single parent, I had been used to remedying , numerous situations on a daily basis. Like for instance, juggling appointments. One child may have a dental appointment, or the other has a parent teacher conference, I'm not feeling up to it, but I push through anyway. Then there's work, I rush my children to the babysitter, and off to work I go. On the way my little one, who was two years old would always cry, because I worked the night shift, and she wanted to sleep in her warm crib. My eldest girl, would have her sisters' diaper bag with blankets, and my son held the book bags for school the next day.

Their sitter would see to it, they got on the school bus in the mornings. I'd pick-up my baby by ten in the morning, and wouldn't see my two older children, until 3:00 PM later that day. Those were tough times for us, trudging through cold winter nights. At the time, I had been working in a residential home, caring for disabled adults. Home away from home, but work and I loved it!

From time to time, I would be asked to work my day off, and would always go in. Especially the month prior to the Easter holiday celebration, because that's when my children and I would go on vacation. As long as my babysitter said it was okay, I'd be able to do a little over time. The only thing that I didn't enjoy, was leaving my children.

When time permitted, I'd find myself standing outside their school yard, like a stalker watching them play during recess. It's a good thing the teachers knew me, or else they'd have different concerns. I remember when my children were new to the school, I couldn't just pop up unannounced. But after a while of working over time, I had to make the school office aware of me possibly visiting.

On occasion I'd sign my children out early, just so we'd get to spend time together, before I'd be off to work. We'd go out to eat, to a park, to see a movie... anything, just as long as we were together. And sometimes they'd spot me from afar, and would charge across the play ground, yelling "mommy, mommy!" As if running for an ice cream truck. I was their treat, and they were mines.

I would be so happy to see my babies. From time to time, I'd be too exhausted to get out of my car. I'd sit there looking, to reassure myself they were okay. And this occurred, even before chemo therapy began. Lord knows, how much I missed them. I'm sure lots of parents can relate. Sometimes it's easier with two parents, not always, but it would help a great deal.

No one sets out to raise their children on their own, it happens but you don't foresee it. Unfortunately that's a part of life. The love I have for my children, wouldn't have me doing things any different. With one exception though, I wouldn't do anything that causes cancer, or any other illness. Like smoking, using certain hair care products, hair dye, eating toxic foods, sweets, certain food coloring, or taking hot showers.

Chlorophyl is in the steam that's released from the shower head, and can cause cancer through opened pores. It's best to replace it with a filtered one, just as you would with the kitchen faucet. Many of you may already know of this, but incase you didn't, it's my duty to make mention of it. And I have so much more information to share with you a little later, on how to make your house toxic free.

You may be surprised at some of my findings. I go into detail of how to spy out toxicity in certain much needed products we've been using for eon's. Continual stress also causes cancer, and many other ailments. There were times, when I had to sneak my children to work with me, and this caused me stress, because I could've lost my job. If I didn't have enough money to pay my babysitter, my children had to spend the night at my job.

I did all of those things, and the end result was my own body, turning on me. It became the enemy, by what I was feeding it, and running it down. My doctor clearly explained to me, that the human body doesn't differentiate, between one cigarette, or one hundred. I was a light smoker for a while. I'd quit, than start again, and had become so addicted, until I asked my doctor for medication.

It was not at all the easiest, but I had to get it out of my system, enabling myself to live a healthy life, and be here to continue raising my children. Following the diagnosis many tests were performed. I had biopsies on both breasts, and absolutely loathed having this procedure done. A mild anesthetic was administered, so that I wouldn't feel, the prick of the biopsy needle. The idea alone, of having tissue removed, made me cringe.

Although painful, it was beyond necessary. After receiving numerous tests, that included lab work, a PT Scan, and other poking, and prodding, I ran! I didn't wait around long enough, to get results of tests that were given, to confirm a breast cancer diagnosis. Which was contrary, to what I should've been doing. At this point I needed to truly grasp what my options were. And found, that I didn't have many.

I needed to get away, from all things familiar. What I did was, put in a request at work, for my vacation. This would be during Easter of 2,006. I made reservations at a beautiful hotel, in Dallas Texas for a weekend. And the day I received my tax refund, my children and I high tailed it out of there, headed straight for Texas! I had heard about, an Easter healing service scheduled in Dallas.

With the faith that I have in God, I followed my heart, and made it my business to be present at the service. So off I went.... On a two days drive, with just my children and I. I've often found driving to be very relaxing, and at the time that's what I needed. Going on vacation, is one of the things that prevented me, from giving up, and gave me the push to get me through, what I was about to under go.

In my element, it felt as if the ground, had been torn from under my feet. But in Texas, no one knew me or the situation awaiting me back at home. We arrived in Dallas, just in time for the Easter healing service. It was held at an immense sports arena, which accommodated thousands of church goers.

All there for two purposes.... In celebration of

Christ's resurrection, and anticipating healing, for whatever illness they'd been suffering. It's almost indescribable, the feeling that came over me. Love, and comfort is as close as I can get, in explaining how I felt, It was awesome! The people who sat next to my children and I, were warm, and friendly.

That whole experience, reminded me of a family gathering. The exact feeling that you get, while sitting around the dinner table, with close friends, and relatives. Which made it all the more special. We were having such a good time, that finding out my test results almost slipped my mind, almost... but not quite. Although I wasn't healed, at the Easter service, a sense of peace came over me. Until this day I still have that calm, quiet peace. I had to stop worrying about everyone else's affairs, and focus on my own. Because all of my life, I enjoyed helping people. From giving advice to a good friend, to helping a friend find an apartment, or a job. I had been the Golden Retriever, for so long, but now it was my turn. "Practice selfishness, "was the advice of a co-worker.

Hate to say it felt good, but it did! I didn't totally zone everyone out, but I began getting used to saying.... NO. That word just rolls off my tongue now with ease, and I don't feel no way about it. Escape from reality also felt great, during my vacation. Not having to report to work, not having to pay any bills, and not having chemo therapy treatments.

That one still didn't sit well with me, but I knew I

had to get started. That's if.... breast cancer was found from all of the tests, I had taken. So I honestly wasn't sure what my fate would be, after returning home. On the drive going, and coming from Texas, my children, and I would stop to eat, and play a little bit. This was part of my own therapy, looking back now, I realize just how much, the trip soothed away the anxiety.

We finally arrived at home, I stepped up on the porch, to see the mail box overflowing with mail. Anxiety began to rear it's ugly head again. Do I check through the mail now, and possibly ruin memories of my beautiful vacation? Or should I wait one more day? I had to gain control, and just open the darn mail already! This is what fear had me do... I went over this in my head, as my children and I were unpacking the car, it was silly.

My life was on the line, and I'm sitting here playing Russian Roulette! I honestly couldn't help the way I felt though. I had never been so fearful, in all my life. This thing had control of me, I didn't like it, it was crazy. I had to actually talk my self into opening the mail y'all! I mean it was powerful! Have you ever been faced, with that type of fear?

Hopefully you haven't, not to that capacity. By then, my two older children, were standing by, as if waiting to run a race or something. Ready for a whistle to blow, or a pistol to sound off clamoring for that mailbox. I just let them go for it, they had to release bottled up energy anyhow, from the long drive so why not. Finally I sat in the living room, sifting through tons of mail, preparing myself for the good news, as well as the bad.

Than there's the red light, on the answering machine blanking, in my peripheral vision drawing in my attention. Okay…. I can do this, I'm thinking to myself. Sure enough I had gotten, two letters of urgency from the surgical oncologist, which read something like, "Dear Ms. McAuley, we've been trying to reach you, your tests came back showing you have breast cancer, at a stage 3, you need to contact our office ASAP, and make an appointment to discuss your options."

Wow! I was stumped, and at a loss for words. But… I was strangely relieved, because now I knew for sure what had to be done. My everything was about to change, life as I knew it, routine, relationships… it all had to be readjusted. The time had come to face the music, but honey… I was in no mood to dance. The next morning, I contacted the surgical oncologists' office, and made an appointment to have surgery scheduled. A nickel sized metal device known as a port, had to be implanted. It was connected to the main artery in my chest, directly over the right breast. The chemo therapy medication was inserted intravenously through the port. I had what you'd call a same day procedure, it really didn't come close, to what I'd assumed it would be.

And that, in of itself was a relief. My sister Tanya stayed with my children, and a neighbor drove me to, and from my appointment that day. Prior to surgery, my doctor had a brief talk with me, almost a semi scolding. He reminded me, of how important it had been, for me to begin chemo therapy, and how his staff were trying to contact me to no avail.

I apologized, he gave me a look, as if to say, hey it's your life. He didn't come off as rude, it was more like, this is what I'd do if I were you. As opposed to running around on vacation, like a chicken with it's head cut off. Let's get started, it's important for you to survive!

I had a feeling these are some of the things he wanted to express, but didn't, he just gave me a long glare of disappointment, or fed-up-ism. He was at his wits end with me, but at that moment I realized, how serious a stage three breast cancer was. I never took anything for granted anymore. Every day was looked upon as if it were my last.

To be honest…. I've had some of the best times of my life, during and following chemo therapy. But to a certain degree, because Lord knows, I don't want to ever, go down that road again. No thanks, that's okay, I can find other ways, to have a good time. Oh yes, I can be a comedic about it now, laugh a little, but at the on set of it all, I was a scared straight, big cry baby.

After fully understanding exactly, what stage three of breast cancer meant, it literally became do, or die! So, I did have options, which were, to either, wallow in the stench of self pity, and point the blame, to everyone for not making themselves available, during my time of need.

Or roll up my sleeves, prepare myself and move on from there. I had to gain control, of the sickness, and all of my other circumstances. Most of the time, I had to go it alone, fortunately it made me cement strong. It was like riding a bull, at a rodeo. I mean I had to wrestle, that thing DOWN to the dirt! Sure... I took my bumps and bruises, before grabbing that cancer by the horns announcing.... I'm the VICTOR!

But... first and foremost, 8 chemo treatments were scheduled before reaching that phase, and eventually I did. I was ready to take the plunge, into the unknown. It took a mixture of sunshine, and rain to grow my garden, of survival. One can't possibly, do without the other. Excessive amounts of rain will drown it out, an over abundance of sunshine will dry it up. And not enough of both, will destroy it. I had refused, to allow my garden to wither it's way out of existence.

On the day that I had the port implanted, my children were with my eldest sister, which meant they were in good hands. She understood what I was facing, and offered to be of help, so I had her support, but didn't want to overwhelm her. After resting for a while, I sat on the front porch, waiting for my children to return from a day at the park, with aunty. Finally, I could see their cherub faces a half a block away. As they drew closer, their bright eyes met mines. We all smiled simultaneously, so happy to see one another.

Like a harmonizing chorus they began shouting mom-my! And gazing upon them, helped to ease my pain. I had almost forgotten about the surgery from earlier that day. They had no idea what mommy was about to under go, and neither did I.

My doctor did explain, usual side effects of cancer treatment, which consisted of hair loss, nausea, diar-rhea, muscle aches, and a list of many others. But I guess, for me, hearing about such things, had to come from the horses mouth. I wanted to know, will I truly be able to continue working? Will there be enough of me left, for my children, or for myself after chemo?

A couple of weeks, prior to the start of treatments, I had an appointment with the oncologist. A nurse sat next to me in the waiting room. Like a dummy I leaned in, assuming she had something to discuss pertaining to my care. Without uttering a word, she reached for a hat, wig, and scarf magazine.

She looked like, and was a nurse, there had only been one thing left to do. Ask this woman, an abun-dance of questions, chancing her moving to the other side of the waiting area, or simply saying... HOW? How are you able to continue working, while receiv-ing treatments? Unfortunately we never spoke, and I thought to myself, well maybe she's a private duty nurse, waiting for her patient to come out? Shortly after all of these thoughts, run through my mind her name was called, and off she went. That answered that, and if she kept working in spite of chemo treatments, than

I certainly could and I did. I confided in a friend not long after the diagnosis, to let them know how serious, my situation had become.

In return, they suggested that I apply for disability, and offered to raise my son. I thought to myself… so that's it, write me off and why not just say go walk out in front of a train. Not to seem rude, but that's how I felt, yea why not… throw me under a bus or moving vehicle, end it all right there, her life isn't worth two cents!

Go ahead throw it all away, no one will miss you and your sick self. I didn't expect to hear anything like that, but that's how I felt. I couldn't accept it, and didn't. God forbid, if that person had raised my son, where would that leave my two girls?

They're a family, a close knit family that I will be here, alive and well to raise. As far as disability goes, I would've just sat around looking at the four walls, waiting on a monthly check? Being able to work had become therapeutic, and I could not bear those thoughts, not yet…. it wasn't over for me! There was a major concern, in continuing to provide for my children. Later on, I'll go into full details, of how taking on a second job came into play, and how forming a shedding list, added years to my very life! From time to time, my little ones had to go to chemo appointments with me, and sit in the waiting room. There were also times, when my oldest sister Tanya would accompany the children. I recall her commenting on how, as soon as the nurse hooked the IV up to the Port, injecting the chemo meds, I fell into a deep sleep.

She had been holding my limp hand, and I didn't respond to her touch. She was very concerned after witnessing that. After waking I assured her that I was okay. We were very close, and although she couldn't make it, to every single appointment with me, she did make her presence known. My sister is hilarious! She behaved as though she were hosting a dinner party, at her house.

Before the chemo treatment was over that day, she had met my medical oncologist, talked with the nurses, and had gotten acquainted, with patients in the waiting room. On our way out, after my treatment, everyone at the nurses station were smiling. She has always been the life of the party, and I relished in just the idea of her, being there if even for brief intervals.

It meant a great deal to me, plus it gave the children quality time with aunty. Following my first chemo therapy treatment, I paid close attention to my bodies' response, and thought to myself, "hey, I can do this, no problem." I felt nothing out of the ordinary, until the one day my little girl and I, arrived home after an appointment that she had. She was fast asleep in her car seat, my older two were in school.

I began to have a sickening feeling inside, that I hadn't ever felt in my life, it was the worst! And I thought okay, It's probably something I ate, that didn't agree with me. The medical oncologist informed me, of how some individuals may experience side effects right away. And others may not have any at all, it basically depended on that person.

While keeping that in mind, I thought I'd be fine, being that I hadn't experienced any questionable side effects, until that moment. So I did the usual... park my car, talk to my baby to try and rouse her from her beauty nap, and she began crying. This went on at least ten minutes, too long.

My stomach was doing twists, turns, and everything but the right thing! Before I knew it, I had undid the whole entire car seat, pulled it out of the car, and went running like a mad woman! Purse in one hand, diaper bag, and house keys in the other, praying.... Lord please let me make it, if even just to the front porch! This way my neighbors wouldn't have the latest juicy gossip, with me in mind.

Witnessing a grown woman having an accident on herself, in broad day light. Thank God, they didn't have the opportunity, I made it! I almost broke the key off, jiggling it around opening that door! Once inside, I honestly did my very, very best in putting my baby girl and that car seat down safely, before zooming to the bathroom!

After feeling better, I quickly freshened up and went to check on my little girl, who had fallen back to sleep, whew! I felt badly, about rushing her into the house that way, she didn't know what had happened. Following that ordeal, I phoned my doctor explaining that I needed medication, to ease the side effects. He had offered them in the beginning, but I was so Miss toughie, with an I got this type of an attitude, and so I learned.

But didn't have to learn that lesson twice though. From that day on I had to wear diapers, and it became a temporary part of my daily life during that season. Potty training my two year old, at the same time, was like a hilarious game to her. It was, oh my gosh! She'd look at me like, are you so serious mommy? You really think, I'm going to get on that potty, and your prancing around in a diaper with more enthusiasm than me? I'd be at a traffic light, just left home, and if I coughed or sneezed too hard, I would say, "uh... kids mommy forgot something," and back home we'd go. I couldn't help it, that had to be.... and it was one of the worst experiences, during cancer treatment.

I managed to get that under control though, and finally taking the needed medications helped a great deal. There were many other side effects to follow, during and after treatment. Some of which were truly, expensive to combat. This is where it would be a true test of my will. And a desperation on my part, to think way outside of the box. When digging deep down within, in search of the needed strength to make it all work, didn't even scratch the surface, of what was necessary to get me over the hump! I mean I had to really bare down, and get to the core of myself, and take on a SECOND job. Over the years I had worked two jobs, many times, but during Chemo that's the last thing I felt like doing.

I had only two weeks, to get out there in between chemo treatments, and all else to beat that pavement, and find another job. Lord knows I did not want to do it. But I had to get something quickly before my next chemo treatment, to be able to pay for side affect meds. I didn't earn enough money, or have the amount of medical coverage to suffice paying for the cost, of vital medications.

Because chemo was one thing, that turned into, taking meds for side effects in which I had no control. Then there were bi-weekly injections, which acted as a shield in protecting my immune system. That particular concoction, cost $75.00 and certainly lived up to the task. It gave my body the BANG that it needed. The glorious side effects were, flu like symptoms.

Although it had been painful, it became a love hate acquaintance, and extremely necessary to the tenth power. It felt as if a wrestler, had slammed me around, or a wild kangaroo, had did a number on me. What did Ms. Toughie do? I took the body aches during the first round, but by the time the second injection was due, I had begged almost on all fours, for my doctor to prescribe pain medication.

On Thursdays, during the summer of 2,006 I had eight bi-weekly chemo therapy treatments. The following day, I'd report back to the oncologist, for an injection. I had been informed from my doctor, of how not to visit any overly populated places, because it might've caused a drop in my immune system. Excessive exposure to germs, could have been detrimental, while having cancer treatment.

My whole life style had been altered, during, and following treatment. For example, going to a mall, movie theatre, church, or restaurants, had to be minimized. That's not an easy feat, for someone who frequented those establishments. On one occasion, there had been concern for the level of my white blood cells. Once I fully understood that maintaining, a low profile was what my body needed, in order to keep it going strong, my white blood cell level improved.

I'd bombard the oncologist, with a ton of questions. I was told by my medical staff team, to ask… and so I did. For anything, especially if something didn't sit right with me, I would say…. why do I need this, why do I need that? What's this, or that do? I'm so sure, my doctor wished his staff never encouraged me to ask questions. e would never say it and chance going against protocol, but I'm certain he wanted to expedite, the treatment process, after having to deal with my queries, and get me out of his hair.

I couldn't help it, oh my goodness, I had entered the doctors' office a royal pain in the rear, they loved me, I know they did! I will say this though, the staff at that medical center, were the BEST! They were thorough, in administering my care completely, in a professional manner. I will never forget, all of the help that I received from that facility, which took them above and beyond my care.

And for this I'm truly grateful!! Again… another topic that will be mentioned a bit later, and will put a smile on your face, as it did me. By then, I had received two chemo treatments, and it had began to show on the surface. My skin changed to a pale grayish, and my eyes looked weak and tired, with dark circles underneath.

Then the occasional dash to the restroom, which had been the first of the symptoms, next were the tresses. I've always had a cottony texture to my hair, with just enough kink to hold a perm. So it was a must for me to use children's perms, that had less potency. Prior to my third cancer treatment, I had decided on relaxing my hair.

This made me feel better, and that became part of my new outlook on the situation. To do something nice for myself, at least once a week, as opposed to once in a great while. Again I was told by my doctor, not everyone losses their hair, I just didn't want to be one of the lucky ones who did. I remember trying to cover up bald spots, pulling a little over here, and there to cover whatever was exposed. Each time I combed or brushed, more hair would fall out.

Eventually my hair begin to change texture, and had a brittle feel like that of a scouring pad. Ugh…. I hated this part of treatment, and unfortunately grew to accept my physical transformation. It came with the process, that I'm certain no one falls in love with during cancer treatment.

I can remember, coming in from work one morning, I'm in the mirror fluffing up my curls, and a huge loch of hair falls to the floor. It scared the crap out of me! That's when I came to grips with my denial. I didn't want any of it though, and had all of those scary mixed feelings. Because I had done everything else, in avoiding the realization of having breast cancer.

By putting on a façade, giving everyone the impression, that I was fine, rock hard strong. I was strong willed…. But I didn't want to have any of it! And driving for two days to Texas, in search of a miracle that didn't happen? It could've very well happened, anywhere at any given time. But no…. I wanted to prove something to myself, maintain some type of control, that I was about to loose. I wanted, and needed my life back. Why wasn't I healed?!

I had been a good mother, friend, sister, a good neighbor… everything was good! Honestly, after all of the hell that broke loose in my child hood, and teen years, I didn't want to go on anymore! And while under going chemo, some how I managed to break through, maintain stability, continue to offer my children what was never afforded me. STAYING POWER, is what I had during chemo! I had to dig deep down and find a way to be still, stop running , and just do what needed to be done and move on from there. I had to do it for my babies, there was no other way.

All throughout my having cancer, they still had expectations of me, and naturally because that's what they were used to. I couldn't just drop the ball and roll out, Lord knows I wanted to! I felt like just taking care of myself, and not bothering with responsibilities.

That included running up to their schools for conferences, rushing them to the doctor when they were sick. I was in no way up to doing house work, or homework and other studies, ECETERA! If you're a parent, you know exactly what I mean. I felt a sigh of relief when my ex-husbands' sister, began doing my daughters' hair every week, God bless her!

I can not write a lie and say we were destitute always, because we weren't. And what began as a nightmare from hades, turned out to be alright. But... If anyone ever asked what had been the most difficult time, I'd ever experienced in life, I honestly wouldn't exactly know how to answer,

I'm so serious! All through out, I had faced some pretty tough adversities, starting out at a very young age. I made it to this point of my life, literally by the skin of my teeth! Garnering bits and pieces, of what I had learned along the way. And to be totally honest... it wasn't half as bad as it could've been. Not to say, I'm this invincible young woman, but I had witnessed some things, I had experienced some things, I had been to the mountain top, and back! Through the trenches, and dark valleys where a child/woman should not go alone... and you know what? I'm still standing... SURVIVING! What else was there to do?! Face every obstacle, deal with every let down, disappointment, and expecting a brighter day my friend, it had to be the only way!

Not meaning to stray, but this next mention, is associated with an illness that I had at two years old. So you may fully understand, the fervor, the energy that pushes me, that jolts me awake, in the midnight hour, or breathes a soft whisper, for me to push on! "Come on Rayshawn, you can do it, keep going, don't look back, it's just up ahead, your almost there!"

My tenacious perseverance, is what's speaking to me. I was often reminded, by my great grand mother Birdie Sweat-Elliott, of how my great grand father, Alfonso Elliott, had prayed a prayer of no return. I have many wonderful true stories to tell, but I will try, and make this one brief. My great grand father prayed, over my limp non-responsive, little frame of a body when I was two years old, and suffering from a disease called dysentery.

The doctors had given up on me, but not Birdie (Mama is what we called her). Lots of tests were performed, to try and figure out how to stop the symptoms. There was nausea, and loose bowels, from what I was told. It was killing me, no one thought I'd SURVIVE. Mama called my great grand father at work, to tell him I was slipping away. When he arrived, he asked the doctors, and nurses to leave the room. With just my mother, mama Birdie, and himself left, he begin the faithful prayer of no return. He prayed that GOD would heal me, and take him instead. I'm in tears, as I'm sharing this with you, and just want you to know that you can make it, through any circumstance! While my grand dad prayed, great grandma said my little hands flew up in the air, and I let out a loud cry, signifying that I was going to be just what my God wanted me to be, HEALED! Healthy and as strong as an ox! I thank God for that day, and times, and years to follow were a miracle. Everyday of my life, is a miracle! Because if not for that sacrificial prayer, I wouldn't be writing, or doing anything. I'm grateful to be here, right now to tell my story!

You may, or may not believe it, but I'm telling you, there is a higher powerful force! And…. As my little body gained strength, my grand dads' became weaker. It had to be about two years after, grand dads' ultimate gift to me, is when he passed away. I missed him calling me Red, that was his nick name for me. I was four years old, and I stood strong at his bed side.

I can see him handing me, an empty cup to fill it with water, so he could take his medicine. I will never forget my guardian angel, that's what he became for me, and I'm grateful, thank you Lord! It's funny now, but when ever I'd be in between foster homes, or visiting Mama's house, once in a while she'd fuss, if I misbehaved. She'd say with her southern accent, "Wooo girl your gran daddy would be rollin over in his grave, if he could see what you done turned out to be!"

I hated it, when she'd say that. Translation…. "My husband is gone on to rest, and left me here, alone with no one to enjoy my golden years with, so you shape up, and make it count!" That's what she was telling me, but in her own way. So here I'am, 42 years later, making it count.

Over the recent years I had to continuously, encamp myself around positive individuals, to soak up their energy. To hold that part of my survival experience, in high esteem. And pray for, but step away from anyone contrary to that, and it wasn't always an easy thing to do, but I would try. I didn't care if it were some of my own family members, I would remove myself from their company, certain ones though. They may not hear from me for a while, though I still loved them immeasurably. I needed positive growth, in all aspects of my life. It took a while for me, in realizing that everyone who says," hey you can trust me" is not always genuine. Often times there seemed to be, an IOU in place as opposed to being there for whatever possible reasons, just be.

That's all that may be required, an ear to listen. With honest feed back, not expecting anything in return. So that's been a difficult thing for me, learning how to trust again. After living through many ups, and downs that were basically dished out, unscrupulously, it's hard for me to trust anyone. Although I'm learning, and it's an up hill journey to where I need to be, but I will not give up.

I will not look down nor turn back, I want to know, and need to know what's up ahead, with out skipping a beat, and I wish the same for you. No matter what your going through, find someone to reach out to. Someone trust worthy, because we're all connected, were put here for various reasons, that I believe. I had to learn to verbally express myself, when something didn't sit well with me. As opposed to lying down as a doormat, to be trampled over in order to feel welcomed or loved. No, I had that thing all wrong, and shameful enough this occurred in my adult years! One thing for sure, I've learned to not throw pearls, before swine. Let me tell you, experience taught me that, thankfully... I'm a quick learner.

I'm very cautious in who I have around me now. They must be healthy minded, and trust worthy. If they hold those two qualities, we'll be good friends. I've wasted precious time on the takers, mis-users, and abusers. Don't get me wrong, I enjoy helping people, but they must show an effort in helping themselves also. As mentioned earlier, I've searched for the reasons as to why, I didn't receive my healing at the Texas Easter service. Why was I healed of dysentery, and not of breast cancer?

Well.... As I begin writing "TILL I GROW" it dawned on me, that my experiences were not meant to be held to myself. Tucked neatly, and safely away, hidden from…. the possibilities of inspiring someone else to move forward. Obscured away in selfishness, and again fear. I clearly understand now, why I drove to Texas seven years ago, and having to come full circle with reality, and face my fears. The cancer was growing rapidly, my healing hadn't occurred, did this dampen my spirits?

Yes it did, but not to the point of weakening my faith. In fact, I felt a sense or maybe an intuition, that something good was on the way! Not seeing with the naked eye, but it was certainly up the road, and it was high time! As I write in one page after the next of this book, and time progresses on I get it! My having breast cancer, was not about me… it was about YOU! That's right, you my readers, I seriously mean it from the very bottom of my heart.

How else would I have been afforded this opportunity, in speaking to you one on one. I certainly would not be able to personally come to your home, or walk up to you… hello my names blah blah blah, I need to give you something, that may help with…. who knows? You may look at me like, "who in the world is she? Miss please, go on ahead with yourself!" Then again, some individuals are approachable, guess it depends on the person.

And…. if your from Jamaica Queens Farmers Blvd area, or Woodside New York, (two of my many home towns) no telling what you may do! You may welcome the conversation, or "get outta here , I don't know you fool!" Or simply walk away as if, not to hear a thing. In any case, it all comes back to you. I can't stress it enough, on how important it is for me to share my survival experiences. I find it a privilege in doing so. God forbid, if you, an acquaintance, or a loved one has/ had cancer, I've hoped to encourage you thus far, and please know that your not alone.

Besides, this world we all live in, is too big to be going through a life changing experience, all by yourself. Be it good or bad news, find someone that will help you to vent. Or invite friends over to celebrate a milestone in your, or their lives. We really should take the time out to love on one another more, as opposed to behaving as crabs in a barrel. However, I say that with all honesty without passing judgement, because I'm also a part of the we.

That's right same goes for me, I'm no better then anyone else, but can be better together. Listen to this, you know how when a fashion statement is made, then shapes into a fad, that almost everybody just has to have! That new hairdo, those five inch platform pumps, flare or bellbottom jeans, remember those? Just as these few items I've mentioned came back into style full circle, what's holding us up, with bringing togetherness back? I've heard people say, "the people in the world won't change, it'll never be as the same as back in the day." which maybe true, to a certain degree though.

If we all took the time and at least began some

where, we can fix things. I strongly believe, that for every problem there is a solution. But most important-ly it starts with each of us. With all of vast technology, folks have just been going with the flow, including myself. And at times I find it difficult in keeping up, with this fast paced way of life. Some of us really need to sit down, and do an inventory, on where to began on how to make this world a better place.

Seriously, there should be no one on God's green earth, struggling to make ends meet. Let alone face an adversity on their own, there are too many people well over capable, to lend a hand. One thing for sure, I will try and do my part as best I can, in making the world a better place. Actually here's my debut, right here and now while writing this memoir! Check!

A Place in Time

DEDICATION TO MOM:

As I move further away from September 25th 1998, it seems as though it all took place just yesterday, the day my mother passed away. One of her good neighbors phoned me early on that morning to break the news. My knees grew weak, and I remember pulling out a chair, to sit at my dining table. Instantly, it felt as though my world had come to a crashing halt! My eyes began to swell as they scanned upwardly, checking the time on the kitchen clock, which hung over the front door.

Not just any clock though, this particular one was decored with clusters of grapes, and a beautifully woven picnic basket, French style. It was an eccentric house warming gift from mom. During one of our many shopping sprees, she witnessed my admiration for the piece, and placed it in her cart. We'd go back and forth, "no mom , we're here to shop for you, get some things for the house, or for Tiffany, and Jahvon" (my two younger siblings) she'd say with a dimpled grin, "no Ray you can't tell me what to do with my money."

And so there we were, carrying on as usual like two children, of course I'd always give in. My husband and I had separated, and It was kind of strange, it took some time getting used to being on my own. Mom chose to purchase the clock, for my first apartment. I didn't know where to began, as far as starting over, moving on. With mom's presence it made my situation bearable, I needed a strong shoulder and that she was.

And I'd give a million bucks for just a glimpse, of one of those moments to actually see mom's illuminated smile... oh God, how I miss her. Parents are truly special, no matter how a child is born into this world, to whichever type of parents, never the less, they were chosen for purposes we may never know. But one thing for sure, a mother is... I'm not quite sure of how to even find the proper description. A mother is like, a warm blanket to snuggle up to, she's the one... when you need that extra push, of reassurance you go to her, she knows. I don't care what it is your facing, she cares. Can you think of anything, you've experienced in life when your mom or maybe even a grandma, smoothed the wrinkles and made it all better? And at times she has a way of communicating to her children without uttering a sound. With just a look, a familiar glance, nod of her head, says it all.

And only that child, and mother understand her gesture, I see that as awesome! Who can communicate with another human being in that way, but a mother to her child. Dad's have that gift also, but not like mama honey! While a woman is carrying her baby for those long nine months, the child is connected in so many different ways, to his/her mother. They can feel mom's emotions, they can tug and pull to signal to their mom that their hungry, or whatever else babies do from the inside.

Well I'll speak for my children, whenever I felt hungry they would be in my belly twisting and turning, kicking and pulling at my sides, they were wild! But—in a good way I suppose. And thank goodness my two younger ones were premies, because I don't think I could've lasted for nine months of pregnancy with them… seriously. While cradling the phone to my ear, I noticed the hands of my beautiful time keeper had stopped. Finally, the tears I held back began to roll and tickle my face.

I can remember shaking my head, and repeatedly saying no. As I got louder, working into a crescendo, my mom's neighbor yelled, "Rayshawn, Rayshawn?! Listen to me, you have to be strong, now hold it together!" She had never spoken to me with such authority! One thing for sure, I quickly snapped out of it, and once again she had my full attention. It didn't dawn on me until my mothers' death, of how much her neighbors held her in high esteem!

That particular neighbor had grown extremely close to mom over the years, and was experiencing her own feelings of mourning. Although she was my mother, she also had close nit friends, which became her extended family over a course of time. It took her death for me to see who her true family was. I didn't understand then, of the expectations her friends had of her. They really loved her in the community. She had wanted so very much, to be a part of a family.

With people who would miss her, or be concerned for her, and she got it. After living in Woodside Queens NY for almost 20 years, she earned her neighbors love, and visa versa. I saw with my own eyes, of how she'd take her time and converse with folks. How she'd counsel them through their circumstances, never judging. Didn't matter if you were handsome, well dressed, cute, or badly in need of a bath… she'd still give you the time of day.

But… on that last one she might've given a firm lashing on how to practice healthy hygiene skills, I'm almost certain of that. She was raw and to the point, I believe that's why she was so attractive to people, because of her transparent demeanor, she never put on airs, or behaved as if she were something she wasn't. What you saw of mom was what you got, basically all the time. She knew people from all walks of life. One person who she'd introduce my sister Tanya and I to, were our Godmother Mariam. It was in the late 70's that we had the pleasure of meeting Mariam. She was truly a blessing, and became an extremely positive roll model in our lives. Even though we had spent much of our infant years in church with great grandmamma , and great granddad our God mother had reintroduced what the meaning of church was. We'd attend almost every Sunday, and had even joined the choir at one point. I also remember joining Mariam along with her own family, on picnic outings, and camping trips. Whenever visiting her we'd have a ball, she'd always operate in faith, and taught us to want to believe in something, someone, especially God. I used to love watching her in church, and how she communed with the other members, she also was, and still is well loved. Her and my mom had their special way of communicating, that they'd developed like sisters.

Mariam would give my mom advice, and would talk stern to her with love and concern. She had taken Tanya and I under her wings, during those years we spent approaching the teen phase. This was before I had been placed in the home for adolescents, and Tanya and I were separated. The most important thing I remember of Mariam, was when she told me of how sometimes you'll meet people, that'll take the place of who's missing in your life. I not only believed her, I searched for it and found it to be true.

We had lost touch for almost 20 years, but when we reconnected , I was so happy to see her and introduce her to my children. I had a mouth full to fill her in on. Mariam didn't know my mother had passed away. I explained what had occurred, and how my mom had two knee replacement procedures, but after the second operation, three blood clots had formed around her knee. She had fallen over her walker while coming out of the bathroom, and died of a heart attack.

Everyone was shocked because mom was so healthy, never sick a day in her life. Always vibrant ready to go! And in an instant, the light of her existence went blank. We were given ten more years, mom and I, to become reacquainted with what we had from the beginning. She was granted enough time to make a mends to severed relationships. Whether the relationships were with her children, or extended family members, never the less we all had time to kiss and make up.

Not long after I moved out, and got married I was there visiting mom, Tiffany and Jahvon, every weekend, as if I had never moved. There were times when we'd get on each other's nerves, and naturally all families experience, a little turbulence from time to time. Like mom used to say, war makes love. Back then, I couldn't fathom the meaning of that quote. I saw it as, if someone's getting on my nerves, that's what their doing, aggravating me or what ever.

However... in time I got it, we as brother and sister occasionally would smack each other upside the head... but nobody outside of that circle better try it! That was the hilarious part, now all the attention would be on that outsider who's causing some type of discomfort. Like they say, there's strength in numbers. And mom always taught us to stand together no matter what, and we do, still. Let me just clarify though, we're not going around beating up the world, it's no fun in that.

But what we will do is stick close, as family should. Always supportive of each other, and will honestly give the shirt off of our backs for a friend in need. One of mom's many quality's that were passed down, and I believe that's why people were just drawn to her. They honestly treated her as a relative. The same exact thing Mariam told me, happened to my mother. She knew folks that were like sisters and brothers, aunts, uncles, fathers, and mothers.

She was blessed in abundance, many times over with a huge family. On the days leading up to her funeral, people would come up to me on the street, and hand me a sympathy card. Every single envelope had 20, 10 five, 40 dollars, it had something in it to offer. Her friends and neighbors giving money isn't what had me wondering… it was the encouraging words they'd express. Like… I wish I could give more, Sandra will be greatly missed, or my ole girls gone, she was a beautiful spirited person.

As I walked through the neighborhood on my way to the local market, I cried to myself, because we had spent so much time frequenting that market. And when I entered I had felt so alone, and began to remember conversations we'd have on the way to the market, or on the way to the mall. Over a hundred people must have come up to me, at different intervals, offering their condolences. It was overwhelming to me, because at those moments I realized how much time, mom invested into giving of herself, and loving her neighbors.

Many of us were taken off guard by her untimely death, but we had so many good times that, that's how I will always remember her. We laughed all the time, about everything! You could not do anything goofy or comedic around Sandra, she would crack up laughing! One day after I had moved out, and returned for one of my routine visits, I began explaining a hilarious story to my mother, and her private nurse. Before I could finish, my mother was in tears laughing, and holding her stomach.

It was a story of how I was driving down a one way street, and stopped at a traffic light. I jumped out of my car to hop over a mound of snow, to throw a letter in a mailbox. All the while I'm thinking I'd make it back to my car in time, before the light changed. Well… I made it alright, with my heels up in the air, and a line of cars behind mines! In NYC I expected to hear horns blasting, and people yelling profanities in my direction, but no.

As I lay there in a huge pile of snow and ice, the other motorists simply watched with a few of them snickering and turning their heads, as if they didn't see my butt hit the ground. And as I peeled my pain stricken body from the snow, I limped back to my car, letting out a cry of laughter myself. Oh yes it hurt something awful, but it happened so quickly, and I guess you would've had to have been there. So… it didn't take a lot to get a smile on mom's face either.

I guess she saw the backside of my coat that was soaked from me landing in a pile of snow. She didn't bother asking, instead she read my facial expression, and pieced the puzzle. Anyway we all had a gut busting time after I shared that story with them. The week prior to mom's death, I had a sad eirie feeling, that I understand now, but at the time I felt like I was mourning before she passed on. We'd call each other every day on the phone, just talking about anything.

Next thing you know… my little girl and I would hop in the car heading to grandma's. During that last visit we were outside on a lovely Indian summer evening, sitting near the front of her apartment building, (her favorite spot)and lot's of her neighbors were gathered around, talking and just enjoying everyone else's company. Mom sat in her wheelchair, I sat across from her, as she propped her leg up on the bench next to me, and my sister Tiffany.

Mom wore a pleasant expression, as she sat there staring at me. I kept quite, and she just kept staring, as if looking through me. It was a look of love I believe, of something she hadn't ever verbalized. Which turned out to be her last look at me, and at the time

I felt it. I didn't know that was the last I'd see of my mother, or her of me, but I felt something awkwardly strange, different. Earlier that week we had a big argument, and I left my house key on her kitchen table, to symbolize that I was not coming back to visit.

We'd go through these silly quarrelsome instances, and wouldn't speak for a few days. Mom would phone me, and leave voice messages, but I'd ignore them. My little sister Tiffany who was 19 at the time would call to try and patch things up between mom and I. And I knew once I heard my baby sis on the phone that it was my turn to respond. We all were so stubborn, but something about my sister calling made me feel like, hey we're all in this together, and now I'm reaching out. To you it may seem so twisted, and it was but this was the way we'd communicate, when a mediator or family counselor were not available. In the end we counseled each other, and that's really how it should be.

And then the whole thing, doesn't turn into a blaring mess that way, when everyone's pulling together. It took many years for us to reach that point, but we did and I'm so thankful. That week before mom passed I had a strange dream of her. We'd always tell each other about a weird dream, and would try to find some type of purpose or meaning of the dream. And trust me, some were pretty interesting an far fetched. Usually she would interrupt with, yelling out to my brother who was twelve, or she'd get a call on the other line, it was always something.

On occasion ,we'd have to carry on the conversation at a later time... like an hour or two later, it was hilarious. We'd be on that phone like two school girls. For once, she was all ears as I began unraveling my dream. Strangely enough on that particular day mom listened, with no distractions of hold on I'll be back, she just got quite. Well In the dream, I walked alone dressed in one of those maiden dresses, like from medieval times. I had come to an opening of a woodsy area.

When I looked up, I saw a huge house that seemed to reach the sky, but there were many houses one atop the other, as in stair steps. I began wallking through the grass and felt drawn to this place, which really was a mansion. There was a black iron gate in front of a wooden door, then out steps my mother. She looked and dressed different, wearing servial clothing. Her skin was so beautiful and clear, and her hair was jet black. All I remember was her walking toward me, then stopped short because the gate was there separating us. She held a black iron key in her hand, that dropped to the ground, picked it up and just stood there staring at me.

We never spoke but were communicating, some how. I then understood that she couldn't let me in. I was so excited while telling my mom about the dream, that her silence got my attention. I said mom, isn't that wonderful, maybe the dream meant you'll be walking again and well off, because you were in a huge mansion. You walked to the gate to greet me! Mom maybe you'll win the lottery or something! All she said was, well maybe. I was so happy, because I believed in dreams coming true, and by the end of that week, she had unexpectedly passed away. That precious memorable phone call, was the last we had spoken. Most importantly, we were at peace with one another. It took me the last ten years of moms' life, to develop a healthier relationship with her. My resentment toward her for not raising me, was dealt with as she helped in being receptive. Which had also proven her positive growth over the years. What helped us get through it, was when we began a new. Enjoying beautiful moments with her and my two younger siblings, were the epitome of family. Getting to know one another again, closed the chapter on many hurtful things of the past. But had opened wide, a path through my garden of life, filled with love for my own children. And all that I was created to be, is enough for them.

Weeding Out

OKAY FOLKS… FOR this chapter I will strategically, do my very best and keep it clean. On occasion we all covet change, I know I do. Before, after, and during cancer treatment, that's what I wanted… change. Careful what you wish for, how about this? Just when I thought chemo was enough, the ceiling caves in, LITERALLY! After arriving home, from work one morning the kitchen ceiling had collapsed! I thank GOD it happened while I was at work, and no one had been home.

The kitchen is the focal point in my family, as well as many other families I'm sure. We did home work, I'd be cooking while the children were just, in and out, snacking or sitting around doing every day stuff. Luckily, on that particular night we were out of the house. There was water, leading to the front door gushing out onto the porch. I called 911, and the fire department quickly arrived, turning off the electrical power. Being homeless was the last straw!

My neighbors were awakened—to a language never thought of, in the history of man kind I promise. Seven years later, I still cringe from the thought of that day. Right there, that right there? Was my cue to run for the hills!

I really could've, to the ends of the earth, and back! Leave my children, my job or anything else that kept me grounded. I was already bald, so there wasn't a strand of hair left to pull out. I sat on the steps bellowing out loudly, "Oh God, I just want to shower and go to bed!" I began to go on, and on, crying out phrases of disappointment, and some newly invented ones. After working all night, it would be five or six hours before I'd get any sleep. That's when I felt like I was done, on the edge, ready to leap into the arms of giving up!

I could not grasp, what the heck was going on, it was overwhelming! After witnessing mommies' semi-breakdown, my children went on with business as usual. They began to nit-pick and tease each other, as if it were a regular day. How could they have been convinced, it was not? Mommy was about to loose it, in the ugliest worst way! While keeping a vigilant eye on me, my eldest daughter, attempted to make peace between her younger siblings. To them... she were speaking, another language anyway.

I honestly had to try and relax, wasn't easy but I managed. I remember us getting back in my car, and just sitting there, for how ever long it took for me to wrap my head around the situation. I thought to myself, why now? Homeless... come on, are you so serious?! Why not six months earlier, or one year prior? I was due back at work later that night, and chemo the very next day. Those particular things were priority, they couldn't wait!

The cancer was still there, and bills needed to be paid, Lord have mercy. I'd invested so much time, into that rental property, and for NAUGHT. Painting, installing new carpet, paying to have the poison ivy forest removed from the backyard, and removing mold. Which I learned shortly after the cancer diagnosis, that mold was also a factor in developing cancer. As the firemen warned me to leave the property, I kept interrupting with, "I could use mops, right?" "No maam,!" the fireman shouted with a stern voice. "How about blankets, towels?" I said. Once they informed me of the enormous hole, in the kitchen ceiling, and how the upstairs bathroom, and surrounding structure could give way, I was pretty much convinced. "oh, okay then we'll just go, I think that's best," I said. Because I was not about to have my children, or myself falling through the ceiling, or one of our beds rolling down to the first floor in the middle of the night.

I didn't even want to think along those terms. My usual stubborn self eventually took heed, and listened closely to the firemen. My children and I watched, as the fire truck and police car drove away. Just in the nick of time they did, because Lord knows I was about to ask, if we all could go home with them. After all, I had been an upstanding citizen, and hard working mother, squeaky clean. My children were pretty much well behaved… at times. We deserved better, at least an emergency resource list would've sufficed. But no, they just left us standing on the sidewalk, I couldn't believe it. Had I been climbing out of the porch window, carrying merchandise, they would've put me up for however long. Feeding me three squares a day, not to mention provide an allowance after release, and halfway housing! Thank God for Jesus, that route wasn't ever taken, it's just an example of stories that I've heard of. Prior to leaving, I sat in my car for what seemed like hours, staring at that house and thinking of the good times spent. Then I envisioned a sledgehammer, crumbled bricks, and mortar, smashed windows, and doors ripped off the hinges! It had been falling apart anyway, why not finish it off huh? I was thinking of all types of things to do to that property, and had to hurry, and get away from there, before being dragged away!

My children and I were living in the home, for almost 6 years. After five years I had spoken to the landlord, of me possibly purchasing the property from him, he was all for it. This is why I had worked so hard, in making repairs in the home. But… they're were too many ,coming in too fast and I just couldn't keep up. What was I thinking? We were then homeless with nowhere to go. Unfortunately emergency aid was not available, unless of course the house had burned to the ground, just as well.

I had also envisioned myself telling the story on the six o'clock news, and the next days news might've read "Family of four deemed homeless, due to a blaze that ripped through an old decrepit rat trap!" One thing for sure, more community services and emergency help would've strangely become available, appearing out of nowhere. I'm relieved though, because it didn't turn out that way. Mostly all of the local shelters were at their limit. Luckily for my children and I… there was enough in my savings, to pay for a week in a hotel.

I had to do what I had to do, and needless to say, my thirst for change had been quenched. Although the months to follow, were truly unexplainably wonderful and we were engulfed in blessings! Though I could not believe, the circumstances we were facing at that moment. Usually there is a calm before the storm, the calm part of it kind of skipped over, yet in the midst of the situation I felt a sense of peace. Not instantaneously, but it came. And honey… I welcomed it when it did show up!

I had to garner the strength, to get me through the WEEDING OUT process. If it weren't for this phase, I wouldn't have survived long enough to tell this story. I needed change, well… there it was! I had been ushered into a course of action, rendered homeless. Later that week after the water receded, some of our belongings were salvaged, and taken to a storage company. I had to hurry, and cautiously tip toe around upstairs to gather some clothing, and other important items.

We were starting from scratch. Finally, space had become available, at a transitional family shelter where we could've stayed for two years, but were ready to move out in four months. It seemed as if, the coin had flipped in our favor, and maintaining normalcy was my focus. READERS?! You would not believe the turn of events, following such a nerve-racking ordeal! Our new home... although temporary, became this long-awaited safe haven, transcending my expectations. I needed a break, and was thinking more lucidly, no longer at a stand still.

I had also trashed all ideas, in having my children placed in foster care, or with relatives. My attempts in providing a place to call home, and stability had failed, but... for a short while. Having my children close to me, was the answer to all of my problems. They were the fuel, that burned the fire within me, to not throw the towel... inside out! My children look up to me, and see this big hero there to protect.

I answer most of life's probing questions, when they're curious. But there's times, I'm just as afraid and inquisitive as they are. I want to know, am I raising them properly, are they happy? Can I honestly raise them, to be successful at the rearing of my hands? Can I mold them into productive adults? Then I realized, yes

I can! They were blessed with a great mom, and doing my best is all they really need, towards a head start in making it in this world. I took a lot for granted before cancer treatment, and that's usually how it goes. There has to be a shaking, a devastation, or a wake-up call, for certain individuals to see the light. And I happened to be one of them. Being strong-willed is in my DNA though, I was a warrior as a child, and had to fight for everything. For protection, for love, for freedom of self-expression… everything!

And after carrying the weight of the world on my shoulders, and being labeled as a ruffian, it became a feat in changing my own way of thinking. Changing how I felt about myself took many years. Cancer treatment brought me to humble beginnings, I don't take anything for granted anymore. My eyes were opened, and my heart receptive, for the new transformation that was taking place, in my life at that time. And no matter how hard I fought the changes in the beginning,

I began to realize they were inevitable. The season arrived for me to let go, and flow with the process. It was like a domino effect. First it was the cancer diagnosis, then dealing with becoming homeless, those two realities tore opened a can of worms, that ate everything away, but for the greater good. At the time I was angry with the world! I was, because I felt I was a good person, trying to live right. Not out there beating the system, or robbing a bank, or selling drugs. I didn't leave my children with strangers to go off and party like it was 2o99, I was a good darn mother, and a thoughtful person in general.

So why was this Happening? I didn't get that part. And don't you know, the light bulb finally lit up in my head, bringing to remembrance of how I did need a change. I must've quietly prayed about it a thousand times, and had verbalized it just as much. All I can say is choose your words carefully, when asking or speaking from the heart. What I should've said was, "I need my feet planted on a healthy, prosperous path, with my soul mate walking beside, or carrying me through the garden of life honey. Those should've been my choice of words.

Back then all I did was complain about what I didn't have, or where I wanted to be in life, when all I had to do was put the wheels in motion. I had it all so very wrong, not realizing that every step I could take toward my goals, would bring me closer. It took homelessness, and breast cancer for me to get it. The onset of a desperate situation is what opened my eyes.

It was like riding an escalator, you either go up or down. As soon as you step one foot on, it just glides you along, and you don't get off until it reaches the next landing. You know beyond a shadow of a doubt you will eventually reach the top, and that takes faith, that takes trust, and it takes knowing. Yes, in the beginning I was stubborn, in denial if you will… refusing medical treatment, and afraid of losing comfortability. Not an easy thing to deal with, but I'd quickly realized what was most important, getting through this particular phase in my life… and live.

In spite of all that had happened, there were still lingering moments of hilarity. And I was at the butt end, of the joke… as always. Everything about me was so funny to my children. From my clean-shaven head, to falling asleep while eating, that too was gut busting hilarious to them. As long as they were happy, so was I. In retrospect, it took the focus off of more serious matters, that I didn't want them to worry about.

I must admit, there were times when I'd been taken off guard, from comments sparsely made by one of my children. I'd never know when, where, or how it would come out, but somehow it did. Like for instance, the day my children and I moved into the family shelter, a staff member went through a list of items that we had need of. My son, who was six years old at the time, impulsively stated, "my mommy, and baby sister wear pampers."

Kids will say the darndest things, won't they? I almost crawled under the table, to hide my embarrassment! He began pointing at my wig, and for a moment I thought, this boy is going to pull off my wig! That's when I intervened to reassure the staff member that we had everything we needed. Guess it was too late to make a first impression huh? I was then that diaper wearing, baldhead , new-homeless woman with the three children.

Everyday after that, when the staff member saw

me in the hall, she'd give me a strange look before smiling. After a while I got used to it. Didn't matter if I was the highlight of the conversation, during the staffs lunch break over tea and crumpets, because honey child... we had a place to stay. That was the important part, that I had a place to lay my head, shower, and could look in a mirror to fix my wig everyday. And not having to sleep in my car. Well... that was the next thing if my hotel and food money had run out, thankfully we were blessed to find a decent shelter.

It seemed like once we left that house, things began to take on a shape of it's own, seriously. And not to play favorites, but okay... there was a staff member at the shelter who always offered words of encouragement. So TYLER ROGERS, yes you were my bestie , at the shelter. Whenever I'd check in for attendance, I remember him asking how things were going, and was I feeling okay? He never seemed hurried and honestly listened, to whatever challenges I had met that day. Always giving sound advice, and meaty suggestions. Instances such as that, really make a difference in a person's life. Just showing a genuine concern, is all it took. That's exactly what was needed during that season. This world would be a better place, if over populated with Tyler Rogers'. He has a wonderful personality, and houses a huge heart... God bless you Tyler! And the positive energy that flowed effortlessly, from the other beautiful folks that were put on my path, is continuously abounding... still. I will always hold on to what I've been given, through meeting people like Brenda and Tyler.

And from time to time, I give it away to someone in need of a pick me up. All of the staff members, were truly compassionate toward my family and I. My rental fee at the shelter was set at $159 per month, $1,400 less than what I had been paying. I finally began to realize, we had turned the corner. Because the circumstances could've been a lot worse.

As mentioned earlier, I'd hate to think what would've happened, if the ceiling in that house, had collapsed on one of my days off. Can you imagine seeing a bathtub, or a toilet in the middle of a kitchen floor?! So... I always believe, that everything happens for a reason. After paying my first months rent, we were escorted to a small bedroom, that had a bunk bed, a toddler bed, and two dressers for our clothing. Almost everyday I had to remind my children that we would be there for a short time, and they'd be in their own rooms again.

My eldest, whom I thought would take it the worst, was okay and understood. But of course it took more convincing for my younger two. We had some really fun times while at the shelter though, especially if I had a day, or night off. We'd turned it into a slumber party, eating snacks, listening to music, telling corny jokes, and waking up the next day with everyone curled up with me. My youngest girl was also okay, she'd just stare at people whenever we'd do activities with the other families. Sometimes she'd bend all the way down in her stroller, almost touching the floor to stare at someone.

I didn't blame her, because it was all new to us. I believe she thought we were the only ones that were living there. That we had moved into a big house of our own, and the other families were imposing, what a hilarious little girl. We had no choice in quickly learning to share everything. And my son always had someone glaring a mean expression in my direction, by blurting out whatever came to mind…. it was crazy! But funny, he had me constantly apologizing to folks, and rushing him through the hallway.

You'd think I wasn't teaching him any manners at all. We were so grateful, and added a little touch of HOME, after all that's what it became. During our four month stay at the shelter, we managed to squeeze some familiarities, into our cozy space which made it a smooth transition. We brought in our own bed linens, and the children had their favorite stuffed animals, and other toys. On occasion, they'd draw pictures to hang on the walls.

My eldest and I, talked about how we were going to decorate, once we moved to an apartment. The whole situation brought on a new feeling of excitement, and it was adventurous, something I was used to searching for. And as a child adventure is a given, they just expect it, but in the form in which we received it was truly unexpected. Still in all we always made the best of any situation, and it cemented our little family bond all the more. I had to inform the shelter staff, of my medical situation, and how I would not be able to check in every day for attendance.

Between Dr. appointments, working 1 PM until 11 PM, then reporting to my second job, from 12 AM until 9:30 AM, there wasn't much time. They had given strict orders concerning attendance, and a daily check in, but surprisingly enough I had their full support. I furnished them with phone numbers, and addresses to confirm my whereabouts, they'd make sure I wasn't pulling one over on them, and I totally understood.

I did have Thursday's off, which were set aside for chemotherapy and hanging out with my children. By the third week of living in the shelter, I had the fourth chemo treatment. During that time, I could fall asleep at the drop of a hat, and aside from racking up parking tickets, I can remember my children and I, returning to the shelter on a day when I had a treatment. We marched into the huge restaurant style kitchen, for a bite to eat. I had began boiling some hotdogs for us, in route to our room.

After changing into my warm flannel pajamas, and relieving my head from that wig, I replaced with a head scarf, I fell asleep. Next thing you know, I was awakened to an extremely piercing fire alarm! Then jumped up running to the bedroom door, to see the other families moving quickly through the corridor, to exit the building. I asked what happened, someone answered, "some DONKEY left food cooking, on the stove!"

That's the moment I remembered the hotdogs boiling. I grabbed my little girl, and clamored down the back stairwell, with my older children following! By then those heavy fire doors had closed shut, but I made my way through heading straight for the kitchen. There was a thick cloud of smoke twirling around the ceiling, and thank God I got to the kitchen just in time! The director of the shelter, gave me a look that I couldn't even began to describe!

The families there were already facing tough times, but homeless on top of homeless... come on now are you so serious? The director was in a mood with me! I just knew she was going to send me packing! Get on out of here, before you re-traumatize the rest of the families! That... was the look on her face. I felt awful to imagine what could've happened, but didn't. But... it all worked out, and she did give me a warning, although not as harsh as what was deserving or expected.

Not long after that episode, every Tuesday evening the local university students, would come in to prepare a huge home cooked meal for the families. Because there were lots of mom's who resided, that were working, or in school. Many of us were beat tired by the time we made rounds back to the shelter, after a full day. So Tuesdays were my favorite days, if I had time to get back. Honestly, I'm not quite sure as to how, I made it through the next four treatments, which took two months.

I was so exhausted, and taking a medical leave from work, and applying for disability, began to sound heavenly. At least I'd have sufficient coverage, to pay for the cocktail of medications, that were taken on a daily basis. They not only helped with side effects, but syphered my energy away. I kept on going though, because in the months to follow, I would not be able to work. Two major surgical procedures were on the agenda for me, back to back... Ugh! At that point I had arrived at the novitiate phase. This segment of my circumstance, would be in comparison to... breaking in a pair of fabulous shoes. You love them—chose to buy them, but it may take a little stretching into, before appreciating them. You may deal with pain, and dis-comfort, but eventually they fit. Until, your ready for a new pair, having outgrown the old ones. The choice is ultimately yours. Either you keep the old worn down one's, which have holes, rips, and tears, or pick up another pair. That's what change is all about, trying on something to see what fits best for you. Go ahead, begin a new! Please don't stay stuck like I did, create an adventure! Dare to do , what you've never done.

Follow your dreams, reel them in! I've never writ-ten a book, prior to experiencing breast cancer, or any experience for that matter. But I'm doing it now... HALLELUJAH! If it completes you, makes you want to shout it, from the mountain tops, than do it! Life is but a vapor, the world belongs to who? You… it's yours! Yes, change was quite discomforting my friend, especially when it had been forced upon me.

But the part of it that was in my control, Well, I'll just put it to you this way, it certainly didn't bring out the niceties, for anyone who made it to my shedding checklist. Through my experiences I've developed a keen mental radar, against negativity. Sometimes it may be camouflaged, but if I see it all the better, if I can sense it… I get it out of my space, and fast! One thing for sure, I believe everyone should have one… A SHEDDING LIST.

Mines enhanced every aspect of my life, best thing that ever happened to me! And if you do have one… kudos to you! I'm a survivor y'all! But in order to truly be that, I had to begin the subtraction of some things. The shedding of a bad habit, bad diet, and the one that was more complex than the aforementioned, was the shaking off of undesirable company, TOODLES!

I ceased with playing the caregiver's role, attentively holding everyone else's needs in high esteem, and not tending to my own garden, the core of me. The real Rayshawn McAuley, was brought to the conclusion, of no longer allowing my significance, to be substituted with the resignation of my own self-preservation. By letting go of certain places, things, and people, I now fill that void with simply loving me. It was almost as if I were in a race, running neck and neck with the doubters, nay sayers, and the haters.

Unfortunately all the padding of my former comfort zone. Finally, never realizing I was miles beyond the finished line, they're were new faces surrounding me. I saw forgiveness, genuine love, healthy self-esteem, optimism, and so many more! I welcome them now with open arms. All along, I had been a winner, without even knowing it! Now that I see the light, I won't allow anyone to manipulate its resilience. Just as a newborn coming into the world, cannot retract back into the birth canal comfortably. I hear that's more of a thorn in your side, than the actual birth though.

Change is a pain, and pain can change. So if you're reading my memoir, please take heed. Don't let fear of an unknown metamorphosis, navigate a path for you. In my expected as well as unexpected events, the unknown, the element of surprise in my opinion, creates adventure. Could change be unwanted? Certainly it can, and usually is but... keep in mind, YOU ARE in control whether you realize it or not. Truth be told, anything you do from the heart can never be diluted by what others may, or may not think of you, who cares?

Unless... it's allowed, that's the only way. Being overly concerned, of what others thought of me, had become a major issue in my growth. I can honestly give a rat's tail anymore, of how I'm perceived now. I've raised the bar, of my self-esteem. This chapter of weeding out, could've been inscribed in my life many times over. But I wasn't ready to maneuver, at this capacity at that time. Hey... better late than never! I was not at all prepared, to split the atom of the indifferences in the company that I kept. They weren't bad, crazy, horrible, folks they were just at a stalemate.

Negatively in a mannequin stance. Not particularly going my way, and once I reached yet another crossroads, I chose to branch off... going solo. Still I have no regrets, I had to open myself up to all things positive, grab unhappiness, and stress by the reins, and ride it out of the way, in full control. Now I see the desired effect, sprouting up and through my garden. I'm not sure if you've heard of it, but GREEN-UP, is a phrase used to describe a plant, coming out of dormancy, and putting on new leaves. By the time, you all get to read my memoir, I will have gone through the green-up stage. I'm here to show, and tell through my experiences, to empower someone along their journey of survival. The new Rayshawn, is exercising an unforeseen boldness... modestly, and sexily y'all! That's right, I'm feeling it now, the newness... for it has been a long time coming.

And although I'm no math whiz... one thing is certain, I nimbly taught myself how to subtract, and divide. Never the less, in a totally different mathematical form. At this point in my life I'm gradually, though selectively, flowing through the adding phase. I'm loving the woman I've expanded into, more than ever before! I can laugh out loud effortlessly, and wasn't always inclined to do so, but now I can.

Feeling pretty light these days, trust when I say, it's a great place to be… considering. As we were settling into our temporary home away from home, I'd put chemo on hold by missing two treatments. The shelter was in a different city, and thankfully my sister Tanya, also lived in the town where the shelter was. To make matters even better, she told me about a woman she knew, that had a licensed daycare in her home.

We were introduced, I examined her credentials as she presented them to me, and I began bringing my children that night. We were blessed, things began falling in place. Aside from work, during that summer, I had to enroll my children into a new school. They all needed physicals for school and the new daycare. This vital portion of my experience, threw my medical routine off. So I had some catching up to do. After getting the children squared away, I begin chemo treatments again, with four remaining.

On the day I returned, for treatment number five, I was greeted by my surgical oncologists' assistant, Brenda. Which I found pretty odd, being that the surgeon's office, was in a different building adjacent to the main hospital. It's as if she were anticipating my arrival. Later on I realized that she was. As I pushed my way through the immense revolving door of the hospital's entrance, I stepped out into a grand lobby. To see doctors, patients, and nurses shuffling about. The cafeteria was in close range, of the lobby. Tucked off to the side, between the cafeteria, and main entrance, was an electrical playing piano. It added a touch of class, with sounds that soothed the soul.

Upon entering, you could smell a mixture of delightful aromas, from the cafeteria while hearing a sweet melody. I associated that, with the times I had visited, my great grandmother mama's house. She was a superb cook, from Orangeburg South Carolina. Waking up in her house in the morning, was like being in a bakery or a soul food kitchen. You could smell those homemade buttery biscuits, and coffee brewing. Mama's strong alto voice mixed with a twinge of baritone would be singing church hymns.

Her strong, authoritative voice, trumpeting throughout the three-story home, was an everyday occurrence. Similar to that of an alarm clock, but less annoying. Some of my favorite cousins, lived there… so I always had a ball when visiting. We'd never tire of hearing mama sing, she was the best! No one ever knew the tools, I'd use to ease my pain. Actually this forum, is the first time I've ever mentioned that. I've heard people say that writing can be cathartic, I'm convinced.

Back then, I never knew, that I'd reminisce on such a lovely memory, to get me through this particular phase. I smiled and waved at the surgeons' assistant, who was in the middle of having a conversation with someone at the admissions desk. She smiled then nodded in my direction. Didn't want to be late for my appointment, so I continued through the bustling corridor. I heard a comforting voice calling out, "Rayshawn!" I stopped to find it was the assistant.

She quickly placed her arm in mines, escorting me to the cancer center. I'm fighting back the tears as I'm writing, because I felt so alone at that time. I needed a good friend, and briefly my shedding list crossed my mind, but trust me… it was brief honey. Because I had no intentions of reverting, kicking up feelings of despair. Guess I needed someone to pay attention to me. Or just listen… to any ole thing I had to say. As we walked, the assistant asked why had I refused treatments?

After I checked in, we both sat in the waiting room. She went on to remind me, of how very important completing the chemo regimen was. All of a sudden, I broke the silence in the waiting room, "We're homeless!" I exclaimed. She handed me a tissue box, removing one to dry my face, and sat there holding me, like I was her daughter. At the time I'd known her a little over a month, a complete stranger. Yet another moment I will never forget.

Finally I calmed down, verbally unraveling what had happened. "My children, and I, had to move into a family shelter, losing mostly everything," I said. She stood up, briefly walked to the nurses station, returning with a notepad, and began writing without utterance. She'd look up at me, then proceeded, quickly scribbling on the notepad. By that time my name was called, prior to leaving she asked me to come in an hour early, for the next appointment, and meet her in the parking lot. I felt as though I had entertained an angel, that's what she was to me. I was feeling more and more drained as the cancer treatments progressed.

And by me having to reschedule appointments, chemo number five was like starting all over. But I had no time to fool around with. A lumpectomy was scheduled for October 26, 2006, and what a busy time that had been. Plan (A) was to have eight treatments to shrink the two tumors. And if the tumors were still visible, Plan (B) was to be enforced, which meant having a lumpectomy.

That consisted of removing the remains of the tumors, as well as surrounding breast tissue that might've been cancerous. If all else failed... Plan (C) was to have a mastectomy, removing the entire breast which I fought tooth, and nail to avoid. And plan (D) through (Z), were to get the heck on with my life! Those are the ones, I was striving for, but still I had a long way to go. Just before chemo number six, I met Brenda as promised. I went inside the doctor's office, looking for her, she came out into the waiting room and handed me an appointment card for an MRI.

Thankfully, it was a reminder that my stint with chemotherapy, was nearing it's end. The MRI was scheduled for the beginning of October 2006. At that time it was around the end of August 2006. Then we chatted our way to the parking lot. After reaching her car she opened the trunk, which was stuffed with bags, and boxes of clothing for my children and I.

Earlier I made mention, of how I had some good times during chemo, well… This was one of them. I gave Brenda the biggest hug, and went on and on with how grateful I was to her. I had been convinced, that there were still good hearted people in the world. God was, and still is so good to my family and I. Shortly after, I left for my appointment with chemo number six. Whenever the treatment was over, I'd drink 2 cups of strong coffee, and hop in my car heading back to the shelter.

My children's new babysitter, would keep them for extended hours on Thursdays. She'd free up extra time for me to rest before I'd pick them up. On occasion, Tanya would have us over for dinner, which helped me a great deal. While dinner was cooking, my children would be playing with aunties' hamster, fighting over the television, or talking their aunties' ears off. As for me… I'd be in the bedroom sprawled across my sisters' bed listening to the hooplaha, before drifting off to sleep.

My two-year-old would find me, and climb in snuggling up with mommy. Each time I'd awaken to my little girl tucked in front of me. She would be lying so close, that I could smell her rose scented hair, and the baby lotion on her skin. Lord knows, I missed spending time with my little angels. Their actions showed how much, I was also missed. I knew I had been doing something right, in giving them the best of me, that was left to give... my heart.

That's one thing chemo couldn't touch. My two older children, begin at their new school, around the same time, I'd endure chemo number eight. The last treatment thank heavens! Although I did have to have one more full year of chemotherapy, but not until February of the next year 2007. Radiation treatments also began February of 2007, and were ended a month later. The name of the last chemo medication was called Herceptin. Which had been given to prevent a reoccurrence, and had less intense side effects.

All in all, I had a nice break before this part of the medical experience began. After the eighth treatment, I was able to quit my second job, but stayed on an extra month at my first. Because the next phase, kind of gave me that extra push in the right direction. I received a letter at the shelter from an apartment complex. And had forgotten completing an application for the apartment seven months prior. Well... the deadline for my response had come and gone.

The notice was almost 2 weeks old. At that time, I was preparing for surgery. Would I be able to relocate yet again? The new apartment, had been an hour away, how could I possibly pull this one off? I began thinking about medical coverage, not being able to work, and also enrolling my children into another new school. Finally I crumbled the letter up, throwing it in the trash can of my room.

I thought nothing of it, but not totally wiping it from my mind. On that particular night, I called out sick to rest. So that was the first full night, my children and I actually slept over at the shelter. We'd randomly stop in for naps on a weekday, or Saturday during the summer months. This was my only night off, for at least the next two weeks, I was exhausted beyond words.

We were all fast asleep, and around three in the morning, my neighbor began fumbling through her closet, scraping wired hangers along the wall. Then she had a heated argument, with someone on her cell phone. I found myself knocking on her door, it flew open and she said, "What?!" "look... I don't want to argue, but you need to be a little more considerate, in keeping the noise down" I said.

All the while, she's giving me a look of disgust, before quietly closing her door. It later dawned on me, that she'd not only had been looking at my bald head, but also the expression of exhaust on my face. Y'all know what my story was, but she had no idea. The degree of strength, it took for me to trudge through chemo... was the same potency, I garnered to go back to sleep, and just let it go.

I certainly was in no mood, for a wrestling match at three in the morning. Sleep deprivation is not a good recipe, when combined with all types of stress, to the 10th power. I'm not a violent person, but I'm only human, and at that juncture I was feeling some kind of wild! Thankfully it was nice, and quiet for the duration.

One thing for sure, I quickly retrieved that housing correspondence out of the trash can. Later that morning I called their office, and was asked to sign, and fax it back ASAP. That's exactly what I did. The apartment was still available, can you believe that! I was the happiest… mama in town! All I could say was, THANK YOU GOD! My family and I, were nearing stability once again!

In a short span of time, I had the MRI which confirmed me having to have the lumpectomy procedure. That's when I put in a request, with my first job to go on a three month medical leave. This broke my heart, I didn't want to stop working and just sit around.

At that juncture, I had worked over 20 years as a caregiver for disabled adults, and also in nursing homes, and was used to holding my own, but my health was a priority. I had to do what needed to be done… and so I did. Finally my medical leave was approved, to began October 23rd, 2006, through January of 2007. I basically worked up until, three days shy of the surgery. It had been scheduled for October 26th, 2006. Everything began moving so quickly, and before long I'd arrived at the threshold, of the next phase of my experience. All that I had been through, from the time of my birth, had prepared me for whatever come what may. God gave me everything I needed on the day I was born. A certain measure of faith, much needed strength, love, and understanding.

Although I didn't understand then, I matured into my wisdom as time moved on. And naturally, with age comes the realization of wisdom, a seed that had already been sown into my garden. So when life throws grapes at you, what do you do? Honey… you make some wine, sit back, and enjoy it! But… In moderation, a measure of wine wouldn't hurt it.

That's right, relish in the moment before the next phase presents itself, because it will every time. That's life, always progressing onward, through cycles of change. It has to or we'd all cease, to exist in the circle of life. I no longer hold onto fear of change, as in once upon a time. "Observe the people around you," my mom would say.

Until this day I do that, but to a more fine tuned degree, especially after becoming a parent, with a fierceness behind it. I pray, that the children God has blessed me with, won't be bound by the fetters, that held back generations of long ago. Most of which were held back, because of their own fear of change. Not all, but too many had dropped the ball, and thrown in the towel.

Perfect example: my mom didn't raise me, she could've. But she was dealing with some hefty fear of going through cancer treatment herself as a single parent. Shouldering the everyday hustle, and bustle of survival, Who knew?! 30+ years later, there I was on mom's old path, which began as the exact scenario, but panned out differently.

Doesn't make me any better, then she. I resisted, as well as tolerated change, until it became me. It caused me, to not give up at times when I so wanted to, Lord have mercy! I was in training, teeter tottering back and forth with this thing, until I got it right. By all means, I'm certainly not the impeccable one, only God is, in my eyes… in my opinion… through my faith.

So when the next phase presented itself, I was able to with stand the unforeseen blow to a weak spot. I may be weak but God is strong, and he never sleeps isn't that wonderful, can you imagine? And… my God never gave up on me. Which brings me to the question of, are you willing to not give up?

Are you willing to pay it forward, to help someone so they can avoid falling through the cracks unnoticed? Better still, are you willing to pay it forward to you? Trust me when I say, I've made that mistake many times of giving much-needed aid to someone before first loving me, which can be a good thing at times, but being that I didn't have the strength that should've been gained from loving myself, I was trampled over.

Loving who you are, allows your self esteem to flow as high as the heavens. That's when, no one can dictate, or attempt in showing what you're worth is because your confident, and you get it! I feel so much passion in this subject right here. For the simple fact that my going through cancer treatment applies to a totally different perspective on life now. Especially of how I view certain individuals. Show me who you are! I hate guessing games… Honestly. Once some-one shows you, who they truly are, they can no longer hide behind inconsistencies. I learned this the hard way y'all. Still hanging in there with a person, going that extra mile with them, after seeing what they were about.

Putting all things Rayshawn, to the side. Neglecting my pursuit of happiness, and at times my own integrity. Now that's a fool isn't it? Not any more… eventually I caught on, sometimes you need to make it all about you, that's right! SOMETIMES though, I'm not constantly going around with an air of, "I'm all that look at me." It's the type of thing that suffices enough, to feel, as opposed to wearing on your sleeve, or posting to your fore head. Once you feel it inwardly, it will naturally show outwardly or anyway you choose. Everything works from the inside out. Like for instance—the lamp, compact disc, or personal computer, you're using to read or listen, to this book … where'd it come from?

It was placed in the heart, than appeared as an idea, in the left brain, which holds intellect, creativity, and thus becomes substantiated. All form a feeling to an idea, to the light bulb in your lamp, to your eyes-balls on this page :). Now that's deep right? I feel like scientist McAuley! Kind of catchy, huh? Back to mem-oir… so now, I'm on to something.

All throughout "TILL I GROW" , I've talked about, survival, paying it forward, change, self-preservation, and last but certainly not least, the shedding list. And guess what beau of a word, comes to mind... it can describe everything I've said, at least in my opinion.

I could be wrong, but it feels so right, you give up? Don't give up now... Okay, here it is! When I went into labor with my children, it was pain like never before! From that pain came life. When someone has survived anything, they're life has been revived. And so on, and so forth. Well for me, everything describes LIFE, it does. I'm so happy to be here, that I may tend to put a little more emphasis on things.

I'm beginning to feel like Paul Revere, rapping on your door proclaiming, "I'm here alive and well, with my children, LORD THANK YOU!" Your probably thinking to yourself, "she is just too radical with it," and you are so right! Most of what I've discussed, you may have heard before this, but... certainly not to this degree... I'm feeling good y'all! That's the beauty of individuality, coming into your own expressing the uniqueness of you. We all have a different story to tell, I pray you won't ever have to tell a story like mines, EVER! I give that to YOU... from the bottom of my heart, a genuine sincerity my friend. So when you go through whatever it may be, that causes you feelings of despair, think about your last test. Bring to remembrance a prior trial, that you over came. For real I'm serious, think of how you got through it, broke through, screamed or cried through! No matter from whence it came, didn't you survive it? But... my question to you is how did you make it out alive? How in the world did you climb that particular mountain, that frustrated you in the first place?

Maybe you've experienced heartbreak that cut so deep, all you could do is wonder... how'd I get here? I'll tell you how, you survived the best way you could, you resurfaced with LIFE! No one on this planet has the power, to take away that in which you have accomplished, not one living soul... and that's real talk all day. Unless of course, you allow it and I believe you wouldn't have that happening.

Especially after over coming, arriving to where it is you'd like to be. It makes so much sense, doesn't it? I know that going through a tough patch, and finally being able to feel and see victory, isn't easy. I'll tell you one thing though, it certainly would be hard as heck for me to allow anyone to pry it out of my hands!

I would fight tooth and nail to maintain, which was the norm all through out my life. Fighting for a place to exist, to just be. Holding onto whatever it was that I had struggled to acquire. What I'm saying in essence is, if you've strived for something, keep your head up. Be it pushing yourself through college, beating that pavement for a better job, leaving behind negativity and not allowing anything to stand in your way of success. Whatever your pursuit is, just keep it moving, and some day you will be smack dab in the middle, of living your dream. Experience is definetly the best teacher, and it has taught me the do's and don'ts of life.

Something's I've learned the hard way, out of my own ignorance. But there's also experiences where I will not have to go through them ever again. It's funny now... but I can remember my dad spanking me when I was younger. Because I was mule headed, thought I knew it all, typical teen. Pops was always calm and collective, but the first time I saw him riled up, is when I had did something.

And why did I have to take it there? Anyway, once my dad got a hold of me, and it only took that one time. All I can remember... after he whipped out his belt and it met my behind was him saying, "don't do it again, don't do it again!" Lord have mercy on me, from that day on, whatever I did to cause my dad to get after me, was never ever done again!

Just recently my dad and I had went grocery shopping. Then he began working on my car, so naturally I had placed his food in my refrigerator. After repairing my car he ate dinner with my children and I, then he went on home. Later on he called me and said, "Ray I'm going to get you, I forgot my groceries at your place!" Right away I got a shiver up my spine, and had a quick flashback of that spanking, that my father gave me years ago! It was hilarious, I didn't mention it to him though, and we just kind of laughed it off. The next day I brought him his groceries, but I was shaken up for a moment there. Oh no... somethings I only have to get clear in my head once, that's all it takes for me.

Which brings to mind an experience, on another occasion where I had learned the hard way. For this particular lesson learned you'd probably say, "big dummy, got exactly what she deserved." Well, after my children and I spent three years, in our new apartment, we could not bear the racism that was prevalent daily. I won't go into full detail, and for me it wasn't so bad, I just tolerated it. But honey, when it came to my children, that was a whole different animal for me to deal with, it was!

I didn't buckle from mean looks, or racial comments toward myself, it took my children coming in from school, wearing a melancholy expression. Just looking at them told it all. If my son had walked in the door quietly, I knew something had been so wrong. If he didn't charge through the front door, after leaping off of his school bus, it struck a cord in me! That's when I would ask how his/my daughters' day went at school? If it had been a minor mishap, fair enough, I'd write the teacher a friendly letter to raise her awareness of whatever had been causing my childs' unhappiness. There was an instance where I'd almost challenged the school district, with a legal confrontation, to be resolved before a magistrate. And rightly so, if an adult threatens a child, that needs to be addressed.

Well it had been on two occassions too many, and enough was enough. Then I began to relate to the world renowned Mrs. Rosa L. MCCauley Parks, who sat and stood for equal rights. My dad is actually the one who informed me, that we may have been related to Rosa Parks. Our last names are spelled the same, (I dropped one letter C out of my name in fourth grade) I had the same trait of tenacity as Rosa, and knowing that sparked a fire in me! But on the other hand, there was such a thickness of racism in the air, to the point of suffocation! We had to get out of there, even for my children to play outside with other children, became challenging. I remember feeling like, if we remained in that environment something would have to change.

Sure I could have fought for equal rights, but really shouldn't have had to. Then I thought, well maybe if we stick it out, my children would be old enough to over look certain things, and just fit in. After a while I had been convinced that, that would've dampened their spirits, having them feeling less of a person. When they are equally if not of more importance, then the next human being no matter the ethnicity, or gender dagg on it!

So we high tailed it on out of there, expeditiously! After experiencing cancer treatment, homelessness and other things, I couldn't bear a court battle over foolishness. Once we were met with this particular crossroad, at the first chance we relocated again. The day following my eldest girls' last summer school class, we had our car packed up headed for GA!

We bid farewell to yet another closed chapter, looking forward to the next. An elderly relative of ours for a very long time, had been asking me to come down and, move into her huge four bedroom home. Although I wasn't sure of the right moment to take her offer, I did promise a visit after all of my doctor appointments, and surgerys had been complete.

Little did she know our visit would end up being a permanent one. My auntie was so happy when I phoned, letting her know we were on the way. She was living alone after her daughter relocated, to another part of Georgia, which placed quite a distance between them. Making it a little difficult in the two visiting one another as often as they wished.

My cousin saw to it that her mom, had regular check ups, and still maintained all of her moms neccessaties. Once I moved in I kind of took my place in helping as much as possible, that is until, my youngest child and I became very sick. My aunties' home had been growing mold, due to a leaky roof.

I remember my little girl and I running high temperatures, coughing constantly, and experiencing excruciating headaches. My aunt and older two were fine. The chemo had weakened my immune system, to the point where exposure to anything made me sick.

Things definitely weren't going according to how my aunty, and I had planned. It had to get better, although not at first. After talking it over with my cousin, she had the roof repaired, then realized how expensive mold removal would've been. It had exceeded my aunts budget, also placing her in a position of re-adjusting her own life.

Finally with much resistance, she had no choice but to move out of her home. Plus there were so many other situations that had her overwhelmed, at that time, that it was best for her to move with her daughter. Which left my children and I homeless AGAIN.

There was no room for the four of us at my cousins', and we certainly were not, and I say that with a capital N honey! We were not about to go back to, the misery in which we had left in the northern part of the USA! So what then, how would I explain to my children? How would I be able to tell them, mommy has failed you guys again?

How in the world did we get back to nothing?! I just knew they were disappointed in me, the one whom they've always looked up to. I was the one, that had been chosen to be their mother. It was me all along looked upon to ensure their safety, I was entrusted with these three human beings lives, and yet again had failed them!

If I were them, I'd want to get far away from someone, who'd constanly drag me through hardships. Some were of no fault of my own, but this one really put their love for me to the test. And if I were them,

I'd never want to bother with me again. Guess what though? My children loved me still!

I couldn't believe how understanding they'd be! It was amazing, of how patient they were... with me. I was reminded of other times we had been displaced, and how they saw mommy working two jobs, in spite of homelessness, and battling cancer, always making time for them. Putting their needs before my own, sacrificing sleep.

Letting them know that, they were number two in my life after God. And I'm telling you, that's a pretty special position in my opinion. Because by me keeping God on my mind during the tough and good times, it gave me the strength to keep moving forward. To continue on with my children, because they needed me.

Just to know that someone needed me, were expecting me to walk through a door, after a long day at work or a doctors appointment, put an emphasis on it all. Knowing someone was eagerly waiting for me, to even return from the grocery store was touching.

My presence had been significant to my children, and it took us being homeless twice, for me to realize it. I hadn't ever known that type of love coming from another human being, ever!

But my children had it for me, and I thank God everyday for blessing my life with them! Before my cousin and I banded together in cleaning out, her moms' house, my children and I moved to a local hotel. At first my eldest daughter was uncomfortable, with having her school bus pick her up and drop her off at the hotel. Which had been understandable, in not wanting her friends to know we had lived there. So I began taking my children to and from school. Not taking the time in noticing if in fact, my son had felt the same. Although he never complained, and probably didn't care much anyways, I just decided on transporting them. Actually, he did make small complaints of not being able to ride the school bus, and cut up with his friends, as some children do. Besides, that's supposed to be a fun time. At three o'clock the school bell rings, and they get to enjoy each others' company, before heading home. I personally remember those days, when I was in school. So missing his school bus ride home, had been a challenge in the beginning. I remember pulling my car into the hotel parking lot, right after my daughters' school bus had dropped a few children off, to her surprise and mines. By the look on her face I could tell, she had been relieved to learn that yes, everyone goes through tough times. And by a few of her friends residing in the same hotel, made the three week stay a little easier.

While my children were at school, I had the unwanted pleasure of getting out there in search of an apartment. My funds were low, and a bi-weekly child support payment was not enough in keeping afloat. And being in the thick of the recession, added more grey hairs, no one was hiring. My many years of experience in the health care field, was a joke!

I had been out of work for three years prior to that, due to having had breast cancer, that kept me from working. So the willingness was there, but there were no jobs. Then I thought, well maybe I will apply anywhere that would hire me, and forget my past work history, with benefits. So I began changing my job search, to settle for what had been available, still nothing.

After visiting and phoning numerous community outreach services, I became so frustrated! The $200 weekly hotel bill had me tapped, with barely enough for food, and to put gas in my car in search of work. How in the world would I get my children and I, out of this doosey?! And after you read what I'm about to say, you maybe feeling like "you know what, Rayshawn deserved every bit of what ever she went through! She put her own self through this situation, I'm done with her! I've got to stop here and say, yes there is a God! Looking down on me, with merciful loving eyes supplying ALL of my needs, every time! Let me please tell you what happened next, you may not believe it! And what I'm about to tell you, many of you may have done all your life.

For those of you who haven't I encourage you to give, or sow when it seems foolish or unnatural, just do it anyway. Before the closing of this book, you'll see exactly why we all need each other to survive.

Okay, what I did next was really not even my own full decision. Well, after dealing with the many frustrations, I had become a grouch toward my children, and the feelings of defeat were about to over take me. I became saddened, and once again met the edge of giving up, and was about to.

It seemed that nothing was working out right. Applying for subsidized housing, didn't help, due to their long waiting lists. The family shelters were packed, and there was a challenge with changing my address, to the hotel which I then found help in doing so. That went well, just when I thought the clouds were passing over, I was told my children had to go to school near the hotel. Me being an honest person, gave my children's school the hotel address, you know, just in case of an emergency.

I guess the other parents at the hotel, kept their mouths shut and moved on. But no, I had to and really I did, have to be honest. Some how, the school worked it out to where I had to pick up and drop off my children everyday, or else they'd be transferred. I had been doing that all along, and just had to keep gas in my car, because their schools were quite a distance. Okay getting back to what I initially wanted to mention, where I said would cause my readers to question my common sense, or decisions that I had made without giving a second thought.

While one door after the next had closed, I became desperate. And during the days of old, when I actually had a nine to five, and had bank accounts for my children and myself, I would give to a charity, or a ministry, to help those less fortunate. My children were also taught to give, and not take their blessings for granted. Although we were down to our last with everything, and the support payment had been our only means of everything, I gave $300 of the payment to a well known ministry.

Leaving $7.00 in my pocket, before the next payment which was two weeks away. What encouraged me to let go of that money, was a supernatural visitation! I remember putting my children to bed, after dinner, homework, and showers. I sat at that kitchen table in the hotel, holding a can of roach spray, looking over my children as they slept, to keep bugs away from them. This had become a daily ritual, I had become so tired, and disgusted with myself, hopeless.

Finally, a few hours before it was time to wake everyone for school, I climbed in bed and began drifting off to sleep. I hadn't been asleep for very long before hearing, "His eye's on the sparrow, and I know He watches me." In my right ear, as I slept as clear as day, a heavenly voice sang that song in my ear! When I woke up to look around, no one was there, it wasn't a dream because I remember checking the time. It was less than an hour that I had fallen asleep! Fear was no where to be found, and a peaceful presence filled that kitchenette room, so powerfully that I felt revived! With a made up mind to continue pushing on! And I will say it right here in my book, of how God was with my children and I. At our lowest, of the low, when we had nothing! Shortly after receiving the next support payment, I thought about those families, who's needs were more desperate, then my own. By me sowing an entire $300 to a ministry, to help others, blessed my children and I tremendously! For every door that had closed, new ones began opening, and at the right time!

We were able to move, into a three bedroom apartment, one week after sowing that money. Letting it go, because it did not belong to me. All that we have belongs to Him, God is still on the throne, yes He is! He makes it possible for us to get what we need. And at times, we're over abundantly blessed with what we don't need. Most people don't even have a roach motel to live in, with a few crumbs on the table. And how about fresh water to drink, or a toothbrush to use?

Or what about soap to keep their bodies' clean, or a pair of decent shoes to wear? When some of us have a closet filled with all types of shoes, and a wardrobe bustling over with clothing! When theirs' people in our world, and right here in the USA, with not enough. All of those thoughts ran through my mind, then I let that money go, as if giving to a relative or a friend. But it had been given to a stranger, and I've found through my many experiences they're the ones who took care of me. When I was sick and had no where to go, a handful of strangers found me and my children.

It may seem weird to someone on the outside looking in, who may have never had a brush with death, but I know where my true help originates, and that's with my God! Whom I will be eternally grateful to! How can I be ashamed of someone, who's not ashamed of me? Someone whom I've never laid eyes on, but will show up, and show out for me His daughter! I have to say it right here, and right now of how my Lord has taken me through, what most may see as bad luck.

All I can say to that is, my Lord went through more than I could ever fathom, yet and still He loves me. And anyone who decides to trust in Him, will have a time of it! So for all the many ups and downs, I've counted it all JOY! Y'all don't want me to start preaching, on the goodness of God! He's performed so many miracles in my life, to the point that all I can do is seek Him out, when I feel alone or afraid, with no answers. My mother is the one who taught me how to pray, and expect results.

She once broke it down, and made it clear on how to reach the ear of God. She told me to talk to Him, as if talking to a live person. Because He is alive in me, and through me. There's no natural way, that I could've made it over the many hurdles, thrown in my path on so many occassions, without a supernatural hand of guidance. And As much as I love my children, I can't honestly say if I'd lay my life down for them, by being nailed to a cross, could I do that for them?

My love is tremendous for my babies, but would I? Could I do what my savior did? At the end of the day, the recession had what ever power, I allowed it to have over me. And once again I had to toughen up, face my fears and move forward. That night at the hotel four years ago, after my angel sang in my ear, my eyes were reopened to matters of the heart. I stopped warming the pity potty, took my power back, once again things began to shift. And my life wouldn't ever be the same. God is still on the throne, Thank you Lord!

Weeding Out…Part 2

CAN'T HELP BUT think of how different my life is, after the much needed transformation. An encyclopedia sized book would be fitting in describing, and unpeeling this banana. I used to wish that my cancer experience, was that of a fictitious article I've read about. Or one better, have you ever awakened from a vivid nightmare, breathing a sigh of relief because as real as it felt, you know it wasn't? Naturally you rouse to alertness, and every day moves you further from that moment… right? Well for me, my nightmare was a reoccurring one, an everyday down spiral. There were days when I would just sleep for hours, and my blankets comforted, and protected me. Hiding me from the sur-realness of the circumstances. There were times when I'd lie to my children. "Mommy's not feeling well today." I'd say. And I wasn't, but they took it as, mommy has a cold or is sick from Chemo. Why not throw caution to the wind?

Just pick up, and leave because I didn't feel up to

dealing with responsibilities. At that point I thought long and hard, about having my children placed in foster care. If only mom was alive, I missed her like crazy. Without a shadow of a doubt she would've taken over entirely, putting a dent in my situation I'm sure. Once I crossed over, into the realm of reality, of acceptance, I was then able to move beyond self sabotage. Move beyond denial, and anything else that had me stuck.

In no wise, did it happen over night, but eventually it did. I thank God for giving me the strength that I prayed for daily. The moment of truth had arrived, my children and I were so excited to be moving, out of the family shelter and into our apartment. My leave of absence began, October 23, 2006, and we moved on that same day. I had the lumpectomy, October 26, 2006.All in one week, without skipping a beat, and had rented a small moving truck.

My sister Tanya, and my children, moved the few items we had in storage. She stayed with my children, and saw to it they'd be okay. Two of my new neighbors, were so very helpful. They offered to drive me to, and from, the hospital after a four day stay. I was an hour away, from my new apartment, but 4 days was too long, not being able to see my children. On the morning of the surgery, I asked my neighbor to let me out a short distance from the hospital's entrance.

I needed to get some fresh air, and clear my mind before surgery. I was nervous about the procedure, but was more concerned with returning to work. For one, I had worked for so many years, and had forgotten what it was like not to. My children, and I needed furniture, kitchen supplies, and winter coats, just to name a few. How would I replace all of those things, with being out of work? Before surgery, the nurses monitored my vitals. The surgeon entered the room, once again clarifying the procedure. He asked did I have any questions?

I replied no, but if only he could've heard my thoughts. "Doc, I'm afraid and don't want to go through with this! Can I have more time to think about it?" Did I really have ample time? I wished I did, but didn't. Although the tumors had shrank, they still could've went in reverse. Growing in size, and out of control. Finally, I got the thought out of my head. My doctor left to go prep for the procedure. Just before going under anesthesia, one of the nurses asked, "Ms. McAuley, is there someone waiting for you after your procedures over?"

I rolled my eyes at her, until they hurt! She had no idea, of how many hours of therapeutic counseling, I should've had on going it alone. I had worked hard, on getting past feelings of alienation, and fear. It wasn't her fault though, she had been extremely patient, and cordial with me, simply doing her job. Once it was over, I awakened in the recovery room, with a sense of relief. All I yearned for, was the sound of my three darlings' voices.

I asked one of the nurses, how long would I be in recovery? She explained, that would be up to me, my vitals, and how quickly I'd wake up. I was given ice chips, to avoid an over load to my digestive system, just enough to wet the pallet. By eating them, it helped to rouse me. What I really wanted, was a good ole t-bone, a salad topped with onions, and my favorite peppercorn dressing. Mouth watering, wishful thinking though.

Before I knew it, I was in my private room, scanning the place in search of a phone. I knew my children were concerned, and I needed to ease their worries. As long as there was a phone nearby, everything was peachy. Right after I got situated, and comfortable I fell asleep. I woke up to call home, and I'm not sure how I got through the call, because I kept dozing from the anesthesia. I could tell, the children were getting frustrated. "Hi mommy, we miss you! Mommy guess what?!" my little girl said. Than my son says, "mommy's not there!" My eldest girl chimed in, with an authoritative tone. "Ma wake up, we want to talk to you!" She said. That's when I woke up, and I'm like, "hold on a minute, are you yelling at me?" we both began to laugh. I honestly don't remember, but when I returned home, Shelaire informed me of just how out of it I was.

"Ma you told me don't forget, to comb my bed, and brush my feet." We had a good belly buster, that day. I was so happy to be home, in our new apartment.

I missed Halloween with everyone... usually we'd go to church to have fun with other families. Well I had been present, but still out of it, and dealing with post operative discomfort. So I really wasn't there at all, let me tell you. Fortunately though, aunty Tanya had great fun with her two nieces, and nephew.

By Thanksgiving I had been up and about, ready to celebrate our first holiday at home, sweet home. Finally a sigh of relief, finally getting things into perspective, feeling normal again, finally a means to an end. I had been on sick leave for thirty days. The healing process had ended, and I began preparing my return to work. Well... wouldn't you know, a week after surgery I received a phone call, from Brenda, the surgeon's assistant. I anticipated her call, would bring tidings of joy, instead she was the bearer of unfortunate news. Cancer was still present, in the remaining breast tissue. I could not believe it, and going back to work kind of slid to the back burner. I was scheduled to have a mastectomy on my little girl's birthday. She was turning four, and we managed a small party the day prior to surgery. We took pictures, and I ate like a cow, because after midnight there'd be no eating. Just before hanging up with Brenda, she told me about a delivery, that was coming to my apartment. Then we discussed the usual do's, and don'ts before surgery. Brenda always had a calming effect on me, like that of a mother. I so needed a mother figure, especially at that time.

Preparing for a mastectomy, began to bombard my thoughts. Okay at least I had a month to recover from the lumpectomy. Which left my breast, looking like one of those cake frosting bags used in a bakery. After the frosting is squeezed out, it's an unshapely eyesore. I hated it, and was almost looking forward, to having that puppy removed. Going from a 42 DD, to one deflated cake frosting bag? No thanks! Less than a week later, a huge 18 wheeler parked in front of my apartment.

There was a knock on the door, when I opened it, two men were standing on the side of the truck. The other asked for me, I confirmed, and signed a long list on his clipboard. Just then, I remembered Brenda giving me the heads up, of a delivery. It had totally slipped my mind, due to thoughts of more surgery taking up space there. Tears began trickling down my face, as my little one stood in the grass beside me, holding my hand. I looked down at her, our eyes met and I flashed a smile.

After seeing my tears, she must've thought I was in pain or sad. But… when I smiled, she knew everything was alright and those were tears of joy! The movers brought in, a sofa, a bed, and a huge oak wood dining table. Dishes, pots, linens more clothing, and some of every little thing we had need of! I asked one of the movers, who was responsible for sending my family such a grand delivery? He explained, that it was from the staff members of Lehigh Valley Hospital.

I went further, to ask how was I to pay for the delivery? They told me it was a donation, even their time. The whole thing was covered, paid in full! This doesn't even begin, to scratch the surface of how my children, and I were blessed abundantly! So... I will attempt... to save my happy praise dance for later on. I'll tell you right now though, God is good! After the movers traipsed, up and down the stairs a dozen times, my apartment was filling up.

I was so very grateful to them, to Lehigh Valley Hospital, and especially to Brenda for sounding the alarm in my favor. Because we had nothing, and were sitting on the floor eating our meals, and sleeping on inflatable mattresses. Sleeping on a mattress was the worst, especially after undergoing surgery. Although we slept, and ate on the floor we had a roof over our head, and were grateful. My children had their own rooms, and I didn't have to hear them bickering over space.

Compared to the one room we shared in the family shelter, our new apartment was like a palace, or mansion. We didn't quite know how to act in the beginning, and knew not to take anything for granted. Anything can be taken away, in the twinkling of an eye. So by my children going through that whole experience with me, will keep them grounded, and I believe for the rest of their lives. It's something they'll teach their children, of how to appreciate what you have. And as they're blessed with more, they'll have it in them to take care of it. The most important thing for me though, is how I've taught my children to share, and give back. I know one thing, they will certainly have some stories to tell my grand children. Which I don't want to see for maybe another decade or two, because I'm not ready to be a grand mother yet, and that's all I'll say about that. Well... after the movers had finished moving all of the furniture, and boxes into the apartment, I phoned Brenda to thank her for helping my family. She'd taken me under her wings, from the beginning. My short-term disability from work, hadn't kicked in and had left me with no choice, but to apply for public assistance.

Luckily it had been approved, then all I had left to do, was find someone to stay with my children before I had the next surgery. By that time, they were attending new schools. My youngest, had begun her first year in head start, so things were finally looking up for us, I just had to get well. I missed one parent teacher conference, but had made it to all of the rest. Their schools were always, made aware of my involvement, and support of my children's education.

I saw to it, that wasn't ever skimped on. Two days before the surgery, I picked Tanya up, she lived an hour away, and would stay for a week on occasions. She eventually relocated to where I lived, although that wouldn't be until one year later. After celebrating my youngest childs' birthday, everyone went to bed, but I could barely sleep and begin drifting, just before my alarm went off. I looked to see the time, it was 4 AM.

They were expecting me for surgery at 8 AM. Before doing anything I said a brief, but genuine prayer. "Lord please take care of my children, while I'm away. Protect them, and all of the little children on the school bus. Please guide the bus driver's hands, amen." I don't know why I used that particular verbiage, in that way, but I'm glad I did. Later on, I will go into detail, of just how significant that prayer became, a couple of days after I prayed it.

Before leaving for the hospital, I went to each of my children's rooms kissing them goodbye, and briefing them with a do's, and don'ts speech. Tanya and I chatted until my neighbor blew the horn, to whisk me off for the dreaded mastectomy. Shortly after arriving at the Hospital, I prepped for surgery, basically following prior procedures. For this one, I had to have a supply of my own blood stored. God for bid if I had need of a blood transfusion.

Good thing there wasn't any need for one, and everything ran smoothly. The only word that comes to mind, in describing my entire experience during that season, is FAVOR! The blessed favor of God. After waking up from recovery, I phoned Tanya checking in with her and the children. As usual I blurted out, all types of babel fighting to stay awake. I was hospitalized for five days and by the third day, I was out of bed, and my nurse escorted me into the bathroom.

When she left, I removed my nightgown to see my chest, and to count the staples that tracked across. By the time I reached 10, I was in tears. The 28th staple count, ended beneath my left underarm area. The surgical oncologist, rounded his way to my room, making sure I was recovering comfortably. I asked him, "so, how are the staples going to be removed?" He answered, "during your follow-up appointment, in my office." I was like, "no seriously Doc, how? Can you knock me out again, because I can't take anymore pain." He laughed, while checking my bandages, replying… "no." After all the poking, and prodding, the tests, biopsies, and Chemo, flip me over honey… I was done! A couple of hours later, I found myself back at the bathroom mirror crying like a baby, and thinking of my children. I began washing up, the nurse wrapped on the door interrupting my pity party. She said, "Ms. McAuley, there's a surprise for you!" I hurried to dry off, and put on a clean nightgown. Immediately after the nurse announced a surprise, I said "it's the children?!" when I opened the door, all three were in my room! My sister accompanied them, and bugged the crap out of my neighbor, to drive them to visit me.

The nurse mentioned how difficult it was to surprise me. I woke up, thinking how their day was going, and they didn't call so I had been a little concerned. Three days seemed forever since I had seen them, it was a glorious visit. Everyone was so excited, as they began explaining a near tragedy. I eased myself onto the bed, after we all squeezed in a group hug, while listening. A huge fallen tree, blocked the school bus route, I almost passed out!

And to make matters more nerve-racking, the school bus runs alongside a river. It brought to re-membrance, the short prayer I prayed three days earlier. The tree caused power outages, and school had closed for that day. Either way, I was thankful it happened, before the bus reached that point. In my life, there has always been a plethora of blessings, that out did the not so good times. To the point where, it's easier to get over hurts, disappointment, and unfore-seen occurrences.

All the pain, heart break, and loss, was covered by a multitude of blessings. Each, and every time, it made me all the more stronger, refusing to throw in the towel. My good friend Brenda visited me, while the children were there. As I'm writing, I'm search-ing my purse for a napkin, to dry my tears of joy. I'm preparing to do my happy dance y'all! Brenda asked me to meet her once more, on the day of my follow-up appointment. It was the week before Christmas of 2006, then I received an unexpected letter in the mail from the family shelter.

Great things began happening in waves, one af-ter the next! My children, and I were invited to come in. We'd been adopted for Christmas, by the shelter, a local university, and the Lehigh Valley Hospital!

All three facilities, had chosen our family to donate gifts to for Christmas! All I had to do was buy a tree. I phoned the family shelter, to plan on stopping by the same day, after my follow-up appointment, and had no idea of their surprise.

The letter from them stated, that the director wanted to meet with me. I thought it had been for something else, maybe I had forgotten something on moving day? I was totally caught off guard. Yes, this was a time when, I really enjoyed my surprise. And having the staples removed, weren't as bad as I thought it would be. The area under my arm, had been numb so I felt nothing there. The brief pain wasn't strong enough, in preventing me from driving.

Honestly, wild horses could not have kept me, from that day! I met Brenda, and three other breast cancer survivors, out in the waiting area. We all took a picture, in front of a Christmas tree, which was beautifully decorated, with colorful ribbons. All the names of the breast-cancer survivors, were printed on each ribbon. Following the group photo, Brenda put her arm in mines, guiding me to the Christmas tree, as she pointed toward one of the ribbons on the tree, I saw my name. What a great feeling it had been, to reach that milestone of finality. Brenda, and the three women left the waiting room, shortly after. I had expected… one or two gifts a piece. You know, maybe a couple of dolls for my daughters. A toy car, or truck for my son, and a hat and scarf for mama, right? Simple and easy, the usual Christmas presents. No sir, it was so much more than anticipated! When they returned they were carrying huge Christmas decorated bags. They had about seven bags, of everything you can imagine, that brought great happiness to my little family! Each gift sack stood about four feet tall.

We were overwhelmed with gratefulness! There wasn't a dry eye in that place. Brenda, and the women hopped in the elevator with my children and I. Once outside, We talked for a short while, as everyone gathered around my car packing in all of those gift bags, and then were off to the family shelter. I kept thanking them, and waving goodbye as we drove away. Again... I didn't expect much at all. I had no idea, our family was even considered for adoption that Christmas, from any one.

The electricity that sparked within, set ablaze an unquenchable excitement! We were greeted, with yet another heartwarming reception, at the shelter. Everyone was smiling from ear to ear, at first I had no idea as to why they were all so darn happy! But then... the director of the organization, approached my children and I, and the university students gathered around us. They began showering us with more gifts, and through tears of overwhelming joy, I began expressing my gratitude.

Someone hurry up, and pinch me, is what I'd been thinking, I couldn't believe it! I felt as though I had sky rocketed 20 feet in the air, and didn't want to come down. It was a feeling that I may never quite be able to describe, and even to reminisce on such an event brings back that energy, it was awesome! I guess the hospital, students and shelter staff were saying to themselves, "we should help this woman, and her children she talks too much!"

It's the truth though, I talked, and talked, and talked some more about the circumstances that over took me and my children, I did. I couldn't keep it to myself, and honestly didn't expect anything, just someone to listen. I needed someone to advise me on what to do. As mentioned before, I had thoughts of asking children services if they could possibly find a temporary family to take care of my children. They never knew what homelessness was, or to even live with a different family.

But when I saw how they worried about me, during those times when I'd be gone a few days in the hospital after having surgery, I knew I had made the right decision. We stuck together even closer, then ever before. And boy oh boy, We were engulfed in gifts, as we set out for an hour's drive home! I felt like a million bucks, like the sun was finally shining my way… FINALLY! It was as though, I were getting married or something, minus the groom.

Hopefully, that will be in the next chapter of my life… ANYWAY! We talked and laughed, all the way home and words cannot describe that day, or that year! Writing my memoir, couldn't do it enough justice. You would've had to have been there, to really get the full extent of it all. I hadn't ever experienced such... love. And to me that said yes, Rayshawn matters also. What her, and her children have gone through, matters to us! We're going to show you love, were going to be the ears you need to listen! We are here, lean on our shoulders for a little while!

You are not cast down, trudging through unnoticed! Grab hold of our strength, of our energy, and we'll carry you and your children to the finished line, thank you God! I was, and I'm still grateful. That's what I felt, the Lehigh Valley Hospital, The shelter staff, and the students from the University, were saying to my Children and I, we are here for you all! And I will never forget that year 2006. I was a stranger, to every single person involved, with the Christmas adopt a family. My continual prayer, is that the GOOD LORD will richly bless them, for the rest of their lives! Because my faith, leads me to believe and know that God was the ringleader.

He allowed all of these things to happen, I personally believe that with all my heart. I've heard through out the years, while growing up, that the good Lord won't put more on you than you can bear, I found it to be so true. Because when my situation became urgent, and I felt like shutting down, and throwing in the towel, that's when help became available. Doors began opening, things began to shift, and it all happened almost microwavable. Looking back now I can see where things could've been more interesting, more dangerous, and more desperate, but thankfully it ALL worked out, for the best. When my children and I returned home, we carried 15 overfilled sacks into the apartment. I remember, like it was yesterday. We unloaded our Christmas gifts, into the first-floor bedroom, which had a queen-sized inflatable mattress. Mostly all of the gifts were already wrapped, prepared to adorn a Christmas tree. Each of my children, received brand-new winter coats, hats, gloves, pants, sweaters, and what seemed like hundreds of toys! There were over $1,000 in Visa gift cards, grocery gift cards, gas gift cards, I mean everything! All that we had lost, was restored many times over, within one month. That bed was overflowing with gifts! Then through my new neighbor, the local fire department had us come in a few days before Christmas, and showered my family with more gifts, and surprises.

We joined in for their annual party, but... there had been one thing about that particular holiday season though, that left me feeling empty. Selfish, or undeserving may be a better choice of words, you know why? For the simple fact that I knew, there were people in more of a desperate need then myself. It may sound strange, but I felt like someone else really needed the adopt a family shower. And it was just that, a Christmas shower for my family, in comparison to a baby shower. Did I really deserve so much? Don't get me wrong now, I'm sure everyone can use a little extra from time to time, no matter what the excess, but I felt like wow! I was sick but got better, we were homeless then had gotten an apartment, I had fallen and got right back up! That's why we were blessed tremendously, because I continued pushing onward, and always thinking of others in some fashion. I'll just say this, my Christmas was not at all complete, until I began giving some of those gifts away. Didn't give all away though I'm no fool honey, we needed some things too now. Or we'd be back to square one, miserable without a pot to... cook in.

But... I gave to people who I thought could use them. So that was another way of paying it forward, to someone in need. I couldn't rest until I was sharing, and caring. Two months after the holidays had come and gone, I was unable to return back to work. And to be honest I needed a break, but didn't expect it in the fashion in which it came. The commute would've become a burden, and there were medical facilities close by, where I could have applied for work but I wasn't ready. I kind of allowed the signals, given off from my body to make that decision. It was telling me to slow down, rest up, and so... I heeded the warnings. For one... I had began radiation treatments in February of 2007, through March of 2007. Radiation went well, though my doctor, had given me a full break, over the course of one weekend. My chest had developed blisters, and a short break helped a great deal. Those treatments were given for five minutes daily.

Besides blistering, I was fine. Then physical therapy began, due to losing range of motion in my left arm. I had developed nerve damage, and my arm had become contracted. At the start of physical therapy, I was prescribed a nerve medication. It helped with uncontrollable muscle spasms, and alleviated the sharp pain, that would shoot up, and down my arm. I had to stop the nerve meds, and work my arm out, loosen it up, and straighten it out on my own. Because the meds not only made me groggy, I also had lost control of both my legs on one occasion. I remember walking down the steps, in my daughters' school. All of a sudden, both my legs stiffened up, from my thighs to my feet. It was like riding a bike, you know the stiff feel you have in your legs, that causes you to walk funny? Okay... that's what I had, It just popped up out of nowhere! Enough to have me sitting on the side of a busy stairwell. I didn't want to fall headfirst down a flight of stairs, for all of my daughters' friends to witness, and God forbid. Besides that, some teenagers don't even want to be seen with their parents, especially in the view of their friends. So I held on, sliding my hind parts down to the step, sitting there until that creepy feeling subsided. I'm sure if I had fallen my daughter would've been so embarrassed.

Hilariously enough, she kept walking, as if she didn't know me. By the time I exited the front entrance of the school, she was already in the car adjusting her seat belt. As I opened the door she just turned to look out of the window. After asking "what happened, why'd you leave me?" she replied, "mom what are you talking about?" I said "you didn't just see me almost bust my butt, on a flight of steps back there?" she answered "uh huh." as if nothing occurred, go figure. Which it didn't and most importantly though I didn't want to be picking myself up off of the floor, with a group of teens trampling over me. By that time, April was quickly approaching that's when I began taking Herceptin. It was a preventative chemotherapy treatment that went on for almost a year.

Thanksgiving, and Christmas were upon us once again, and nothing remotely came close, to the previous year, but I will say this, I was even more grateful to be alive cancer free, celebrating at home. After giving my body almost a year to heal, I had another surgical procedure. It was called a Trans abdominal Myocutaneous Flap, short version? Tram flap... it also sounds better, doesn't it? Now with the Tram flap, it felt as though I was recovering from a C-section. I wanted a normal looking breast, and this procedure was totally done by choice. I met with a plastic surgeon, who showed me numerous photos, of how I wanted to have my breast shaped. Finally I chose a photo, and we went with that. Secondly, during the procedure, my own stomach tissue had been used, in forming my new breast. And for my female readers, you know that unsightly pouch, that some of us are blessed with after giving birth? Yes that's the one...

well I had it three times over, complemented with those lovely stretch marks. But after my tram flap, everything was tight, and right honey! Although much pain was endured, I healed in time for the summer of 2008. Everything I wore, fit as if I had never given birth. I began dating again, and just enjoying the new me. The Tram Flap was scheduled for, December 11, 2007. It's funny how the surgeon's seemed to conduct my procedures, during the holiday season. Healing from surgery, was no picnic just before Christmas. And the day following the Tram Flap, the nurses had me walking the halls. Doctor's order's of course and it helped, because I couldn't stand upright. After returning home, I kept practicing walking, and using my stomach muscles. One thing for sure, I healed better in the winter, than I did in the summer.

The perspiration agitated my stitches, and my incisions would get itchy while healing. I walked around with a damp cloth, the summer I had the right breast reduction. But... for the Tram Flap procedure, my stomach had been sliced open, from left to right. It was pulled up, along with a detachment of my navel. So... walking or anything remotely close to it, I did not want to partake in. But I had to, the hospital staff were prepping me to go home. And my begging for temporary private homecare, was to no avail. I told my doctor, please don't send me home like this! Please, my children will eat me alive! How in the world, would I be able in keeping up with them? Thank God Tanya had been available, to stay with the children and I for the first week. I'm not sure how we would've gotten by, with out her. There were no worries of cooking, or getting my children off to school that week, she did it all! Boy, did we miss her on Christmas that year!

At that time, I had come to another level in cancer survival, during my weeding out phase. The holiday blues crept up on me, thoughts of Christmas past with family and friends lay heavily on my mind. I felt alone, and saddened because of Tanya's absence. Spending holidays together, was so much fun. Taking pictures, playing games with the children, and staying up late nights watching movies. And the cooking? Forget it... When my sister and I get in the kitchen, you'd think you were in a five-star restaurant... seriously! A gift inherited from our great-grandmamma. Though it wasn't too bad, because a few months later she relocated to where I was. So it all worked out, and my children and I loved every minute of it. I had been dealing with depression that was camouflaged with sleep, and anything else I'd use to cover-up. But on the night of Christmas eve, in 2007 it all finally came to a head.

I was awake listening to carolers on television, trying to get comfortable. My four-year-old, was fast asleep on the sofa, I sat upright across from her in a recliner. My little girl loved sleeping with me, but after I had the Tram flap, that wouldn't be happening for a good while. My first night home after surgery, I remember throwing my comforter on the floor, and rolling out of bed, just in time to make it to the rest room. So to avoid crawling on all fours again… getting in and out of bed, I purchased a fluffy recliner. That's how I slept for three months. My little one went into a coughing spell, choking in her sleep and I jumped up! Now mind you, I had glue textured stitches, from the right to left side of my stomach. Not to mention, the JP drainage tubes. They were also stitched into my stomach, on either side, with one in the pelvic area. A JP tube is like a long straw, made of thick transparent rubber. A mechanism used to monitor blood loss, and the drainage of blood clots. I had to empty, measure, and document the amount of blood flow, every couple of hours.

As time progressed, the bleeding is supposed to stop, and it did. So… as I dove into rescue mode, literally those CPR and life support skills kicked in full force. I had annual trainings at work, repetitiously for years, so I knew exactly what to do! Thankfully my audio, and visual senses have formed a heightened sensitivity, to life-threatening emergencies. As I quickly motioned toward my little girl to stop her from choking, I somehow tripped on the carpet. The whole apartment Shook, once my knees hit the floor, and the worst pain pulsated through my body. I felt my stomach pull on the sides, stretching those stitches and tearing at my inflamed navel. What did I do? I turned my little girl onto her side. Not only to stop her from choking, but to avoid crying like a baby in her face, startling her out of her sleep. And I had a long good cry, right there while on my knees, Lord have mercy! I began thinking of that whole experience of cancer treatment. I'd calm down, and cry some more. I asked God to give me the strength, to do what needed to be done. Because for one year, following chemo, three surgeries, and being homeless, had thrown me into a depression. I had been so engulfed with staying alive, keeping it moving, and maintaining my focus.

That Christmas eve night of 2007, all of what I'd been holding in was released, and I had to weed depression out! I was the victor! Not the pitiful victim, and yes I lost a part of me, but being able to spend the holidays with my children, was the epiphany of Joy unspeakable! That had been the main reason, as to why I felt it best for me to continue working. After purging myself of depression, it felt great! Having a good cry every now and then, is refreshing mentally, physically, and emotionally. It got me back on track, and right on time to truly enjoy the holidays with my children. Once again I got up, and didn't stay down! I dusted off my knees, and continued on my path of survival. Everyday became better than the day before, more then what I could ever imagine! And I guess it had to, because I made sure of it!

There was no room for dwelling on the unfortunate times. I will say this much... I use those experiences to continue surviving. Surviving and reaching back and uplifting someone, through the telling of my story. Not at the beginning, but when the moment was ripe, I had been tremendously blessed with meeting great people. Whom later on became my family, they crossed my path for a reason, when I needed them most. It's so true of how we're all connected, in some kind of way or another. Strangely enough, all of those people who came into my chidrens', and my life... I haven't seen or heard from. Some of them I've tried to contact, are no where to be found. There's maybe a handful that are still working at the facilities that helped my children and I.

This confirms it for me that, they were in my life just for a season. At the proper time and place, when I was destitute for real. Not knowing which direction to take, but thankfully I took it one heart beat, one step, one thought, one day at a time. Isn't that beautiful... provisions were made and we didn't even see it coming, It just happened! As one door had closed, so much more was opened to us. Whenever I hear of, or meet someone who's going through Chemo Therapy, or has over come, I make it my business to share my own experience if time permits. And if I'm preoccupied with doing something else, guess what? Whatever it is has to cease, when it comes to offering what I've learned, in prevention and possible alternatives. Reminding them of how they can survive, if they desire. That's all it takes, the need to want to push on. You might say, well what if the persons' in the last stages of an illness? Or maybe the doctors have told the individual, there's nothing left for them to do?

That my friend, is when the individual should refuse to go down without a fight! In my own opinion as long as there's blood flowing through those veins, a way must be found! And it's there if you look closely enough, seek and find. And seek some more with all costs, until the answer materializes. Until your satisfied, and restoration has returned. I had a friend who recently passed away. There was no way I could have contacted him in time, although another friend of ours knew how to reach out. A matter of fact this particular friend allowed skepticism to take over, which left my hands tied. And I don't hold them at fault.

For one, I'm not God, nor do I in any way claim to be a physician, nevertheless, there are websites where you can read testimonials of others who have used cancer treatment alternatives. And this was in various stages of breast cancer, lung cancer, cervical, and the list goes on. All through stepping, and thinking outside of the box. There are folks who have taken a chance, and put away fear of maybe a change of their diet, and other ways to flush out toxins. I never said organically grown, or super foods is a cure, for an illness as devastating as cancer, but why not give it a try? Just like for instance, when a mechanic works on a vehicle. And let's say... the owner hasn't a clue, on how to do the repairs themselves. He/she may not know what the heck's going on, they just know of possible deadlines, to be met.

The customer needs to get that thing fixed expeditiously, to get on with their work week, or other obligations. So the mechanic performs the process of elimination. If he/she's a good mechanic, they will attempt everything in getting to the core of the issue, for the customer. Nine times out of ten, they remedy the problem by working at it. Picking apart every single bolt and screw, finally reaching that point of aha! I found what's wrong, here's how we resolve it. He won't ever gain his customer's trust by forfeiting, nor will he have a business. So why not use the same energy in possibly saving a life? Anything and everything material, in no way should hold more value than a LIFE. When my friend passed away, my heart ached so badly because I didn't get the opportunity in relaying my message. This same message that I vowed to deliver to you all. Where there's a will, there's a way.

Sometimes we don't want to hear maybe this will work, or possibly give that a try. Yes we all have rights, as to whether or not to follow doctor's orders, as well as taking someone's suggestion into consideration. But from what I've researched over the past few years, and have put into practice, has opened my eyes. So much precious time has been wasted, in getting this vital information from here to there. From me to you, so it's being presented to you now, and is ultimately up to you in how to take it from here, or not. I only wish I'd known what I know now.

I'm sure you've heard that before. Man I wish I had that information way back when. Or, how come no one's ever told me this or that, sounds familiar? I also mention natural remedies for combating any type of cancer. I use my past circumstances, and what worked for me to spark interest in that person. Because people want to know of alternatives, to not only save them wasted time and energy, but to also save them some hard earned cash. Cancer treatment is expensive, even for the elite. I'm not exactly sure of the costs for surgery and cancer treatment, but it took me having to bust my chops on two jobs, to be able to afford medication for pain and side effects alone. And for the most part from my own experience with using natural herbs, after the fact... I find most of them living up to standard Expectation, and guess what? They're a lot cheaper then taking the traditional route. And lots of folks will decline throwing they're eggs in one basket. I honestly don't blame them, but sometimes you'll be surprised at how taking a chance, doing research and asking around, can help.

Sowing & Reaping

AS MENTIONED EARLIER, I don't know what I would have done, if I didn't have the care team that came into my life when they did. They saw an opportunity of making a difference... and I'm so glad they did. All of the time they sacrificed in giving of themselves , will always be special to me. Because they could have just did their jobs, get paid and go home. With no obligation, in forming a support network, especially with out getting paid over time, I didn't even think about that. But they did... from the many conversations of encouragement, to having my family adopted for Christmas. To holding my hand, assuring me of how my situation was going to be alright. That made the difference and made my survival walk bearable, at times when I couldn't see my way through. How would I have gotten by, with out a helping hand, or hands? It took a village, It took sacrifice of a strangers time, to reach back and help me out of a pit that I was sinking in, it took love.

Imagine if you will, but just for a moment... don't stay there too long though. Think of yourself taking a loved one, or a friends place who's receiving cancer treatment. You come in from a hard days work, feeling awful because of a chemo therapy appointment a day prior. Depending on their ages, your children may or may not be willing to pull together as a team, in helping you get dinner going or run a few errands. In order to get it done, you result in doing it yourself, pushing and squeezing your energy you had in reserve to do it all again tomorrow. If your married, then use the same scenario for your husband/ wife. No one truly gets you, because they don't know what it's like to walk in your shoes. They don't understand that you may have one foot in the grave, and the other out. Nor do they want to face they're own fears of possibly losing you. Because after all, mommy's / daddy's are forever, right? And thank God this is only hypothetical, because everyone isn't this way. But really... what would you do, if faced with a terminal illness... God forbid? Would you call a confiding friend, to talk you into feeling your best self? Would you curl up in a corner, sulking? Or maybe you'd want someone trusting, understanding, and loving to come and check on you. Wouldn't it be heavenly to have a home cooked meal, at the hands of someone else? Honestly, who'd reject someone else's slaving over the stove? That's if you can bring your stomach to catch up with your mouth. Because some people experience major nausea at the site/smell of food during cancer treatment. Sometimes it's best to have a care taker, or friend prepare your meals in advance, from their own kitchens, trust me it does help. One thing I didn't experience was loss of appetite, I never turn down any type of food.

That is, except for okra, I don't care if it's made with pure gold! I will not touch it, fried, tossed in salad, boiled, or baked no thanks. But I did have nausea from the aroma of smelling certain foods while they cooked. At any rate you'll need some type of assistance, somewhere along the line. Or maybe it'd be nice to have a break from your children, where you can regain peace of mind, gather your thoughts. You could also do nothing, just exist. Sometimes that could be a good thing as well, it's really what your up to doing, or not. The choice is yours, and the world would be a better place , if more of us really reached out to help someone who has fallen by the way side. I know for a fact, that I've been guilty of taking others for granted. I have… even my own health for that matter. As with any garden or growing thing, it will need planting / sowing to gain a harvest. The process takes time, just like with any other. Before ever planting seeds to a garden, you must first know what you'd like to have in your garden. It's up to you as the gardener, as to just how much of a harvest your EXPECTING. Then again, if not much love, care, and quality time is spent nurturing your creation… well we all are aware of what may happen… nothing!

Not a thing, and that garden will shrivel up, into a crisp, returning to the ground un-revivable. And folks, all this chapter of sowing & reaping is about, is just my personal advice. And I say personal because I had walked in my own shoes, to come to a place of survival. I know first hand what it's like to be with, and without. My survival has also taught me of how to deal with people, and how to consider they're feelings and opinions. Like for instance what I do with my oldest daughter now, instead of telling her what to do, I just give her my best RAW advice. Because that's how adults should approach one another, out of care and concern. But with honesty, never pushy or aggressive, just easy flowing advice. So I'm not telling you, "you'd better get in there and help out." Or yea that's right you better give your brother, or sister a hand right now, or else! "No, not in a million years will I have you feeling that way J. As a cancer survivor, and survivor of a myriad of other life altering situations, I'm only giving you my opinion. And there's no harm in asking for what you need. This could be for anything your heart desires.

One vital part of asking… is giving though, or sowing on fertile ground. It doesn't have to hold a hefty price tag. Not at all… you can give of your time, by visiting someone whose sick, or in prison. Or even help an elderly person who's immobile. If planting and sowing is executed in an un-selfish manner with honest intentions, it will some how multiply it's way back to the giver. I've tried it and it works! Once you've mastered that, trust me, someone will cross your path someday, with eagerness to help you out of a circumstance. As mentioned before, another description would be to... pay it forward. So when your time of need comes a banging down your door, and it will... you can repel it especially if you had paid it forward. Which runs parallel with saving for a rainy day... cha chang! Good things will come chasing after you, and you may have forgotten a good deed you've done, but the universe hasn't, God is who I call Him. In all due respect I'm not certain as to what your religion is... but I feel there's a higher power out there. At least that's my own take on it. And it has boldly shown up in my experiences, on many occasions.

Especially when I had no control in helping myself. I'm talking desperate times, which called for desperate reactions. First off here's what you do God forbid, if you know of, or are close with someone facing a health crisis:

1. keep in touch often, to let your special someone know you're a vein in they're support network.

2. Offer assistance if you notice they're struggling in some type of way. Some people may not have to, or wish to be verbal in what's going on, at times it'll show. So here's your chance to step in and make your presence known.

3. Offer to carpool, or chaperone your loved

one to, and from an appointment. Not only are you allowing them time to rest, in the passengers seat, you could be saving their lives. For real, because chemo, and radiation treatments zaps the energy, and the patient wants to sleep afterwards. And I remember the feeling I had, after chemo and having to drive to work, or home following a treatment. I honestly put myself in danger, and could have gotten pulled over for a DUI. Because I knew I shouldn't have been driving, but... had to. So this is a biggy, please offer your help wherever possible to make your loved ones' life more pleasant.

4. TAKE CARE OF YOU... which is just as important as caring for your loved one. You will not be able to do anything in aiding someone who's sick, if you began a down spiral of self preservation. So rest up and take it easy when YOU can.

5. Tag team your loved one... make it a group effort, or a project. Let's see who can love on our patient the most, right! It may sound comical, but I'm serious! Gather a bunch of people who's all in common with the individual who needs assistance from time to time. You can even make a schedule, for instance, Sally and Sue will stop in to check on Lizzy, on Mondays and Tuesdays. Mary'Jo and Billy will drop by

on Wednesdays and Thursday's, Tyrieka and Tyler may check in on Fridays, and Saturdays. How ever it's worked out, the individual who's under medical treatment will be so grateful.

6. Continue until that person is back! Until they can manage the basics going solo. Once they feel up to easing into their independence, I'm sure you'll be the first to know. Try calling that person when their up and about, they may not even answer their phone, and may be so happy with getting their life on track, who knows.

Or they may always be available, especially if the shoe was on the other foot. They'll remember how you stuck closer then a brother. You were attached to their hip, you were the shoulder to lean on, the ear to listen, the heart that opened for them, putting their needs before your own. And trust me when I say, you will reap what you sow, every single time. And how about forming a fund raising group? It really depends on the overall feeling of the person who's not well. They may or may not be able to work, and may be toughing it with keeping up with bills. Let alone the cost of cancer treatment, or any surgical procedures, it could run in the thousands. Unless they choose a different route, and are trusting in alternative cancer care. Like with using natural herbal/homeopathic remedies. The natural way of combating cancer, which can be costly but… is much less expensive, than that of beginning a cancer treatment regimen.

It's certainly worth a try, especially for someone who's retired, and is tapping into their life savings. So in this instance, fund raising is the way to go. I had the pleasure of presenting cancer treatment alternatives, to a cool group of folks. They were holding a yardsale fund raiser for another relative, who had need of paying left over bills due to cancer care. I had told them a portion of my survival story, and shed light on alternatives. They also sold and served a wholesome meal, while we talked. I've heard of many different ways of conducting a fund raiser. For this particular one I played a part in sowing a seed, and it made me feel like… I don't know, like the queen of Sheba I guess. It was a great way to spend my Saturday… and besides I love being in the company of seniors. Listening to their stories, taking in their ideas and seeing things from a different perspective. After all that's what got them, to their life's lessons. So I listen with an open mind and heart. Any opportunity I get in sharing my story, I take it and run with it! Leaving my victim well versed, in all things survival.

Miracle Growth—
In Full Bloom

YES! IT'S OFFICIALLY over y'all! I'm standing up for yes this year! I'm saying yes, to new beginnings! Yes to selfishness, but... with good intentions. Yes to all things positive! Yes to reaching new heights! If for any reason, it doesn't aid in my growth, then I don't want it around me. And I mean that with all seriousness, from the uttermost bottom of my very heart! I've learned, that in order for me to truly live my dreams, and carry out my goals, I need to be in the company, of like-minded individuals. Just as sure as spring follows winter, and summer follows spring, we all have seasons in our lives. I've grown so far from the Rayshawn I used to be, that I can't imagine it any other way. The fetters of alienation, fear of change, of depression, and lack of self-esteem, have broken loose. Now I'm free! Free to be the best woman, that God designed me to be. Didn't see it before my past experiences, but after being pushed to this point, where I am right now, oh boy do I get it! When I look in the mirror, to see the new Rayshawn peering back at me, she looks different, quite cheerful. With a fierce boldness, she has the look of a warrior, but with love in her eyes. Those deep dark excruciating scars of despair, have faded.

The scars that brought about, her fiery journey of survival, are dissolving into the sea of forgetfulness. No longer having to linger, snatched away from it's dwelling place, un-resurrected. As I valiantly travel this new path, I'm harvesting the goodness that grew from the seeds sown, during my storms. As my children, and I move forward we hold in our hands potent seeds, carefully sprinkling them, over fresh rich healthy soil. Needless to say, the torrential downpour has my garden in full bloom. Growing up, and outwardly to the east, to the north, south, and west! All along my journey, I had always given thanks to my creator. First of all, for being a father and mother, to me. By strategically placing those individuals, on my path to fill the chasm, that had once held the missing links... my parents. I've met some undesirables along the way, but other's that I've been blessed with meeting, have made lasting grounded impressions upon me. And to show my gratitude as I'm writing this memoir, I'm paying it forward to you!

My story of survival, has been created to empower my readers. I'm certainly not the only breast cancer survivor. There are hundreds, of thousands from all walks of life. Maybe they've gone through cancer treatment, or has a loved one battling it. Whatever situation you are facing right now, throw out thoughts of defeat, If you have any! Castaway anything that's holding you back, from reaching your mark of enjoying your life. Throw out ideas of giving up! Then I want you to do this dear friend... you shake the dust from your banner of survival! That's right hold it up high, and declare I am a survivor! I'm not dead but alive! I have a purpose here, I'm not finished yet! I have family/friends who love me! And if you don't, seek out new ones! Those who didn't mean you any good, before your steps toward survival, certainly won't be well wishers on your road to recovery, hot dog! And I don't set out, to offend anyone. You decide for yourself, what's best for you.

You don't have to listen to a word I've said. But... If you know what I know, if you've been where I've been, you'd keep a shedding list handy. And begin your math equations, of subtracting and adding. Not saying to cut everyone off, that you've ever known, I'm merely sharing my personal experience with you. I tell you this much, my shedding list had brought some things, to the forefront. Mine eyes, have seen the light. And if a person's own ignorance, doesn't blind them enough, they'll see how to patch things up, and fix it. And they will, that's my prayer for you. You need strong healthy relationships RIGHT NOW! Not years, months or even minutes, I'm talking now. Because as

we all know, time waits for no man. Develop relationships with someone, who understands what you're
going through. If you are, or know someone undergoing cancer treatment, I hope my memoir has lifted
your spirits. I pray it has brought you, peace on your
journey through your garden. All throughout "TILL I
GROW," I've used phrases to depict a garden. It repre-
sents nature, and can sometimes be grimy, or smelly.
A garden also brings forth beauty, with pleasant aromas. I compared my life to a garden, though withering
at first, it has blossomed with the proper nourishment.

As in life on an everyday basis we may experience
the beauty and the un-pleasantries. Sometimes where
oblivious as to which direction to follow. If you look
closely enough, your own path to take will appear. And
once you've reached, the end of that path, search for
another. Continue moving in the direction, leading to
your goals, and aspirations. And then what? You look
back, in view of your garden, with innumerable seeds
that you've Sown. Then take in all the splendor, that was
produced from your hands. Beware though, try not to
linger there for very long. There's nothing at all wrong,
with revisiting where you've come from, especially the
good times. Overindulgence of anything is no good,
but a brief look back every now and again helps with
growth. It will remind you of how you've strived to over
come. Just keep your head up, looking over the horizon
for whatever, your expectancy maybe. A sharp focus, is
what brought me to this point, of my life. As mentioned

earlier, I've always had a hankering for reading, writing, and telling stories when I was a child. Once I became a single-parent, my priorities were not the same, taking the focus off of my first love, a book.

The healthcare field was number two on the list, of my favorites. I kind of got, the best of both worlds so to speak. The first part of my life, I put my hand in someone else's when they were sick. If I said I was going to work or fill in for someone, I was expected to show up. People were dependent on that, my word. I took care of various types of people and it was very rewarding. The way I saw it was, I'm going to spend time with a relative, not some stranger. Because I conditioned myself, to treat each individual like how I'd care for my family. I loved my job and it showed, always. Which in turn was extremely promising and also helped me along with growth. Now for this part of my life, I'm living my dream of being an author, screenwriter, poet and a playwright. I get to tell stories of interest, that I've created, how cool is that?! It's as if I found my soul mate, and I've happened upon, what it is that I should be doing. No longer, pushing my aspirations to the side. Please don't laugh, this is my new title in a nutshell, are you ready? Okay here it goes, I am a cancer surviving, author, playwright, screenwriting, poetry flowing, chef style—soul food cooking, sexy mama! That's what I am y'all, and a happy one too! Just thought I'd share it with y'all first. And I say yes to reaching for the stars, and getting on with it, it's time!

Nurture Your Garden

NOTE: ALL OF the information included here is totally, YOUR choice, if you decide on using. So please don't say, "Rayshawn advised me on changing my diet, to try this!" And you wake up, the next morning with one eyeball larger than the other, or one leg shorter than the other (pun intended) you know what I mean. It's all up to you, to ask your doctor questions, and at your local health food market, pertaining to supplements and proceeding with your best judgment. Now, we all may be aware of causes of cancer, and I've listed a few here. But where does cancer come from? It can be derived from the very air we breath, as well as various foods, and drinks. Like for instance excessive alcohol drinking, can be a culprit to getting a cancer diagnosis. Although I've read facts on how drinking, a glass of red wine daily is good for you. Another is salty/fried foods, which not only cause high cholesterol, but may also be responsible for a variety of cancers. Who doesn't love dark toast, or their red meat cooked well done? I've learned while browsing these sites that I'm about to mention, of how integral it has become, in eliminating various toxins from the diet. Sadly enough… that's the way that most of us have been eating and living in general, filling up on toxins.

Although, there are certain exposures that we simply can't help, the ones that can be helped, we'd better get on the ball, and make a turn around before another 10 years. Five years is more realistically speaking. In hindsight a great deal of what I've learned, after a breast cancer diagnosis breaks my heart, but may be of some help to you, I pray. If only I would've known, why didn't I hear of that sooner? What an awful shame, girl I wish I had known you were ill. You could've had an alternative, to chemotherapy didn't you know? Unfortunately those were some of the things, I've heard after all was said… and done. At the time, I had no idea there were treatment alternatives, but after seeking I found. There's also certain organic foods, that if consumed on a regular basis, can flush toxins out of the body. We all were born with a certain amount of cancer cells, but without a proper diet, those cancer cells begin eating and growing. So changing the diet is imperative. Many of you are possibly aware, that having an alkaline acidic diet, will help decrease toxicity.

Factually speaking, there has to be a healthy balance, in our blood's PH at an alkaline level of 7.365.

Your probably saying "well, how can I obtain an alkaline acidic diet?" I'm so glad you asked, because here's a website that you may find enlightening, www.alkalinefoods.net. After reading through this site, I felt like I had graduated med school or something. So please, check it out in your spare time. I also found a list of root vegetables, that have a higher level of nutrients, then any others: cabbage, Brussels sprouts, carrots, horseradish, cauliflower, turnips, and beets. Another super food is spinach, which is packed with vitamin k, fiber, and strengthens your digestive system. Fresh garlic is one that enhances the cardiovascular, as well as the immune system. Which aides in combating other ailments, or diseases. Garlic also helps to filter the liver, and lowers the blood pressure. As you can easily see, certain specific leafy greens, and other strong nutrients can do one job on it's own. But... with all the needed minerals, vitamins, and nutrients working synergistically, it can create something powerful!

Placing YOU—at the helm of your own health! Putting you in full on control, of what's really best for your overall being! Why not You?! Because honestly... isn't that what we all want? To be living our lives as healthy as we possibly can, increasing energy levels, extending longevity? What's not to like about that? Personally it took me a while, and from time to time yes I get weak. Adapting to eating healthier, after spending so many years eating what I wanted, as opposed to what my body needed, can be challenging.

And just because it doesn't happen over night for some, doesn't mean it can't happen for others. That by the way was my excuse, at first. I would say things like "oh I will start tomorrow, or I will eat more greens next time, it can't be done over night." How foolish was I?! For one, it can happen over night, and two, with much discipline. Folks it is doable, you can change anything about you at any given time. And that's at the pivotal moment when your ready. So it's up to you, as always. On alkaline diets' site, you'll find intricate details on just how important it is, for us to have the proper PH balance of alkaline/acid. I've also learned from other sites of how, cancer can not thrive in an alkalinized vessel, as well as one filled with oxygenated cells. Acid can also come from numerous, healthy and harmful consumption of foods, drinks, and too much cruciferous veggies. It can seem a little contradictory, but there is a such thing of over doing it. Like the old saying goes, too much of anything isn't good for you, and it's true. Because certain vegetables can do more harm than good, if consumed too often. And this may pertain to anyone who may be having issues with high cholesterol, and diabetes, or who may be taking blood thinners. What I did was add an internet search, for veggies that have the unwanted opposite effect. You can always double check, in obtaining clarity. Because just as well as there's super foods, to boost your overall health, there exists others that may not work well, if enjoyed on a regular basis. One thing is certain, cruciferous veggies will supply the body with the much needed nutrients, to maintain a strong digestive system.

On www.livestrong.com you'll be able to search for exactly, what one needs to know about cruciferous veggies/fruits, herbal smoking cessation, dieting, exercise, and developing a healthier life in all aspects. Their site is filled with tips to get you in a better place with everything, in keeping you as physically sharp as you need to be. Did you know that certain fruits are high in antioxidants? And how antioxidants are cancers' worst enemy? Those cells that were exhausted, from chemo can be revived after all, by a regular intake of herbal supplements, and antioxidant rich foods. To be honest with you, herbs can be a little tricky, as the aforementioned, so it's best to do your homework. Ask at your local health food market when concerns arise. If there's a particular herb that strikes your interest, simply search it on the Internet. You'd be surprised as to what you'll find. Also seeking advice from a licensed holistic practitioner would be wise. What I've been collecting from the internet, are informative articles, that always have an experts advice on a particular herb or super food. And they'll have available to you, those super foods, or herbal supplements' unwanted affects listed. For example, a vitamin regimen during chemo therapy may have to change, or stop all together, depending on the patient. And from what I was told by my doctors during chemo, was that cancer can feed off of the vitamins, which can be alarming.

As mentioned earlier, always ask questions, and then ask some more. This way you'll know exactly what type of diet, vitamin, or any other health regimen, is best for you. Which reminds me of a health scare, that occurred in my life earlier last year and thankfully it was just a scare. I'm no health expert, but maybe after hearing this particular experience, it may be of help to you or a loved one. Around January 2012, my right breast had developed a rash. At that time, other issues were going on which caused my stress levels to soar. And stress alone, is liable to cause all kinds of ailments. Swelling had also formed in my right breast. After doing an internet search, I found those symptoms were that of breast cancer. Because when I had been diagnosed almost seven years ago, the only symptom that I had, were two lumps and pain. Which were enough in letting me know, something was so wrong. I didn't have a rash, or inflammation of the breast.

So this time I wanted to confirm, and learned that it could've been. One thing for sure though, I refused to see myself sick and torn apart as before. I saw myself intensely finding a way to help myself, and not rely totally on a traditional approach. And said "oh no not again!" And I meant NOT AGAIN! After relocating I had been waiting for my health coverage to begin. Honestly, I didn't want to get hit with a huge emergency room bill, although that was next on the list. I gave myself two weeks to a month, to see a change in my breast. In the meantime though, I got on the Internet and entered a search, for herbs that MAY kill breast cancer... THAT SIMPLE.

Seven years prior, not only did I not have access or time to research the Internet, I didn't know, but now I do! Anyway... I was fuming when I found various herbs, and supplements that MAY be able to combat all types of cancers! Some but not all, can be taken in unison with Chemo Therapy, if a patient is more comfortable with taking that route. Personally, I would've opted for both the Chemo regimen, along with natural herbs. In my case the chemo not only shrunk the tumors, but it also weakened my healthy cells. For that outcome alone, I'm certain that I would've chosen natural, as well as traditional treatment. Reason being that, the organic method would've strengthened the weakened cells. And the healing phase following treatment might've faired differently. Hey, the more you know, the more you grow. Knowledge also TRUMPS the cure my friend, always! Okay... So I happened across this website: www.mynaturalmarket.com, which advertises the most powerful organic products you'd ever come across, also www.gethealthyagain.com is another. Through get healthy again, I ordered an herbal supplement called Zormus. This particular supplement, not only aided with clearing the rash and inflammation of my breast, it also removed arthritic pain in my hands and knees. When I mention all of the herbal supplements and organic websites, folks are not quite convinced. If any of the healthy natural websites I've mentioned in my book were not legitimate, trust me I wouldn't in no way waste your time. This is serious good news here, I have tried and still use many of the remedies I'm sharing with you. And let me tell you... I refuse to regress to the old way of eating, drinking or to the same hair and skin care products, I had used for years. What else was there back in the day though? Everything was chemically based, for microwavable results, am I right? To tell you the truth there are lots of businesses who are also catching on. Striving to provide their customers, guaranteed decent products, so that's always a good thing.

Copious amounts of natural healthful remedies, are within our reach right now. Folks this is a totally different type of animal, I'm talking about here, that does really exist on how to combat almost any ailment, sending it reeling in reverse. And I can't stress it enough, of how you'll have to take a look see for yourself. We as humans were never meant to clutter our vessels with so much garbage, to the point where a person needs, more poison to ward off the culprit, but simultaneously destroys what's left of the healthy cells. Well not 100%, because if a person who's been treated for cancer, catches on in time they can revive damaged cells by simply beginning an herbal supplemental regime. This has to be a daily ongoing routine though, in order to get expected results. The amount of supplements used at the start, should be taken moderately, to really get those weakened cells back into shape. As time progresses, from what my research on natural herbal supplements revealed, you can scale back. But try and keep it going for the first year. This way your body will keep those powerful nutrients in reserve, incase you miss a day or two.

There's also what you call the dieing off reaction, which can cause an individual uncomfortable side effects. From what I've read about and had experienced first hand, is that it's best to begin natural supplements in small quantities, gradually ease your body into getting used to your new diet. And as mentioned you can increase or decrease your intake of natural supplements. But always begin with low dosages. As with anything newly introduced to the system. I would compare using natural supplements, to an exercise class. Your stretching muscles you haven't in years, and when you wake the next morning, you feel it everywhere! As you continue, let's say,... possibly every other day, your body gets used to the pulling and beating that you put it through. But then again, everyone's tolerance is not the same, as others.

You may not have any negative results. Again, discuss with your doctor before taking, and bombard your local natural food market staff, with as many questions you need, to increase your awareness and comfort. It's so important for you to be at ease, and to have the freedom in knowing what may be best for you. A word of advice, immediately after steaming your cruciferous vegetables, it's a good idea to pour off the excess water from the pot, to remove any impurities that might have stuck around even after washing. This is something I do all the time, and believe it makes sense. There's no way you'll be able to get rid of all pesticides, from simply rinsing although steam cooking them, may be just enough to discourage an offset to the thyroid gland, as too much of an intake of cruciferous veggies may do so. I also ate fresh kiwi fruit, three times a day. Which is best just before rotting... I know, I know, it sounds disgusting but that's where my research of kiwi led. The kiwi fruit is more potent, with higher levels of good old vitamin C, the longer you allow the process of ripeness. Which calls for a little patience, or you can purchase them already ripe. What I do is feel for firmness/softness, then I choose. Then I ate fresh leafy watercress vegetables raw.

Sometimes I allow the watercress leaves, to sit in 8 ounces of bottled water closed tight sealing in those nutrients. I did this for two days at a time. Just let it marinade in the refrigerator, hold my nose and then I drank, UGH! It's nasty, it stinks but is good for you. From my research of watercress, I learned that many years ago, the Greek nationality, native Indians, and herbalist used watercress to ward off diseases. Watercress is also rich in antioxidants, and contains a very high level of vitamin C. Strawberries and blue-berries are two power fruits at the top of my list, rich in antioxidants and vitamin C. The thing about berries are, that it's best to eat them in variety, instead of sepa-rately. You can enjoy your raspberries, blackberries, strawberries, and blueberries in one sitting. Just pile them on all at once. Eat them as often as you can, until there streaming through your nose, eyeballs, and ears, they'll also exit the other end with easeJ. I'm telling you, after I did this for a few months, my right breast cleared up! I had blood work performed, once my medical insurance began, and everything came back excellent, no cancer! Just to think, all it took was com-mitting a little time toward research, and changing my diet. But… the ultimate test, was to follow through, and make a significant decision on sticking to it.

That's the thing, actually taking my health serious-ly enough, to want to remain healthy. Often it takes as much time in over coming a habit, as it did in devel-oping it. Which may not be true in all cases, but man oh man please do not flash a chocolate chip cookie in my face, because it will take determination, of a made up mind to resist. I'm keeping it real, with all honesty. Which brings to mind, natural sweeteners, by any chance have you heard about those?! Let me tell you, oh my gosh! I've found a way to cheat, but with-out added calories and higher glucose levels. Instead of baking those fattening cookies, muffins or brown-ies as in days of old, you can try this, agave nectar, molasses, or xylitol, all natural healthy sweeteners. Your local wholesome/health food market should carry those low calorie sugars.

One important factor about Xylitol is that, it's a great natural sweetener that doesn't promote cavities. And can be found in the ingredients of most sugarless gums. You'll be able to gather more information while browsing www.xlear.com. This website lists numerous healthful details, in which Xylitol can be used. From what I've read, and noticed in my own usage, is that Xylitol, helps to level blood sugars, and prevents cavities. It's a wonderful substitute for regular sugar, and tastes great. Xlear.com even has a listing of candy with Xylitol in the ingredients. Please check out www.goop.com, where you'll find organic products, with everything your body needs, in keeping it in optimal shape. Their site is bubbling over with all types of information! Here you'll catch a glimpse of, international travel, latest fashion, and lots of other mind-boggling finds. Goop also has an abundance of delectable recipes, that will blow you away! Once on Goop click the JOURNAL icon, then hit the GET icon, scroll down to the photo for Natural And Organic skin care. You'll be amazed at your findings, which are organic everything! From natural nail care products to, toxic free make up, organic skin exfoliators, natural hand sanitizer (which I'm adding to my personal list) a must have natural anti-wrinkle skin care product, organic baby care, and the eco-friendliness goes on. A definite eye opener, that you'll have to see for yourself. Another site where they list wholesome, scrumptious recipes is, www.whfoods.com. It will leave you scientifically sharp, with what not to eat, as well as what to add to your dinner table. Whfoods has helpful articles on salmon, and other foods, that may raise a brow, or two. And you must be extra selective, when purchasing salmon. I'm sure your aware of the two types of salmon? For one, it's extremely good in promoting a healthy heart, with it's richness in omega 3 fatty acids, the good fat I should say. Although the wild salmon is rated a better choice, there is a flip side. Unfortunately wild caught salmon carries higher levels of metal, as opposed to the farm raised brand. I absolutely love salmon, but going with the omega 3 capsules maybe someone else's preference.

Thankfully they're available over the counter, at your local pharmacy, and health food market. Other fish that are packed with omega 3 is, lake, brook, and rainbow trout. Out of this trio, lake trout comes in first, in measuring highest omega 3 properties. Whfoods is a non-profit foundation that has scientific accuracy on a variety of harmful not listed here. I believe you'll enjoy reading the many helpful tips while whipping out your cook ware, to try your hand at one of their recipes. Now that we've gotten a mouthful on what actually enters to please the palette, and keeping it healthy, how about we examine, other ways in maintaining YOU. I mean really going all in, and all out, for the caring as well as the keeping of you! The first half of Nurture your garden, was introduced to shed light on developing healthier eating habits. This second half of the chapter will equipped you in various forms, on how to spoil yourself with organic skin/hair care products. And ladies, In no way do I intend on discouraging those biweekly manicures, and pedicures but… beware! I had tried a nail salon, twice in my entire life,and felt I had deserved a little pampering. Why not, after running to work, then standing, and walking for seven or eight hours.

Keeping up with our children, and their school activities, who wouldn't feel like a little something extra, in melting away all of that tension? So, to finally treat myself, I went to get my nails done up! They were beautiful! Then I found myself going again, because I so deserved it, right? And that pedicure, with the leg and foot massage, Lord have mercy… was out of this world, I was sold! Shortly after my second appointment of spoiling myself, I was infected with Candida. Candida is a fungal infection that plagued my nails, hands, and feet to no end! It became a nightmare of the worst kind! I had developed a complex, and didn't want to wear sandals in the summer, and would always hide my hands. They looked like they belonged to a crocodile, it was awful! And If the utensils, that are used aren't sterilized properly, they will have bacteria growing, as with anything else.

This can cause Candida infection, and is treatable

with a topical and oral antibiotic, but… in the early stages. Unfortunately, with my busy schedule at the time, I allowed It to grow out of control. By the time I made an appointment with my doctor, I had gauze on my hands, and bandages wrapped around my feet. Now I'm aware of organic nail salons as well, can you believe it?! After trying the antibiotics, the end result? It didn't work for me, and got worse. I had it so badly, that I don't think I'd even trust an organic nail salon! Although there's very few that I found in my web search, they do exist. Personally, I don't ever want to go near anybody's nail salon. Whenever I see one I get flashbacks, of the horrible oozing of my hands and feet, and those painful blisters, that became a thorn in my side. After a certain amount of time, the

Candida entered my blood stream, which made it difficult as heck to get rid of. What really threw me off, was when my doctor discontinued the antibiotics after a month. Just when it had began relieving those excruciating symptoms. Due to the fact that the medication could effect ones liver, blood work is mandatory every two weeks. I figured the Candida would eventually go away. That was before ever having been diagnosed with breast cancer, at least three years prior. That's when I learned of how candida may contribute to a cancer finding. So… I did a little search on the Internet, and honestly this particular product can be used for the interior, as well as the exterior physical make up of you.

It can work wonders for your overall being. It was a diamond in the ruff to find: www.aloelife.com, and their toll free number is, 1800-414-(ALOE) 2563 to contact customer service. Recently I had the pleasure of speaking with, Karen Masterson Koch, CN.. Karen founded Aloe Life over twenty years ago, and I'm thinking to myself, where the heck was I?! She shared a portion of her sharp expertise with me, and it blew my MIND! Karen Masterson is a woman, who knows her stuff. We had such an enlightening conversation, as we discussed the Aloe Life juice. And let me tell you... after drinking Aloe Life in it's concentrated form, the Candida fungus went away. Didn't happen over night, and to speed the process along, I also used Cand Eilm plus-repair combo, which I found on www.candida-yeastinfection.com. The site is affiliated with www. gethealthyagain.com, that had been mentioned earlier. Whenever my Aloe Life juice runs out, I have a supply of Cand Elim. When I use both products synergistically, it's powerful stuff! What Cand Elim does is, destroy viruses, bacteria, and kills candida. More importantly, this product gets to the root of candida literally, preventing re-occurrence. I also use Nymsar Elixir from candidayeastinfection.com. Nymsar soothes the die off side effects, and any other possible allergic reaction. Which can be nausea, diarrhea, and muscle aches. I began seeing results, between two weeks and a month, I looked and felt like a new person. Sleeping at night came easier, and I was more alert during the day.

Why does this sound like a darn commercial? Something I hated listening to, unconvincing mumble jumble. But it's true... if I hadn't been plagued with that miserable skin fungus, I wouldn't had believed anything about Aloe Life, or candida yeast infection products. That's what hindered me, and gave me second thoughts on darkening a threshold of a nail salon, the fear of contracting something. Now that I'm aware of what can be used in ridding one's self of candida fungi, I want to spread the word on how to get leverage on this thing. It doesn't affect everyone, however, proceeding with caution is one's choice.

From my own experience, I've learned that Aloe Life, not only flushes away candida, it has many other strong properties. Such as detoxifying the digestive system, as well as strengthen the immune system. Because from what I've read, candida latches on to the intestinal wall, upsetting the digestive system. Gi-Pro completes the Cand Elim repair combo, and actually works to heal the intestinal wall, by replenishing lost nutrients. I had no idea, that a low functional system, can cause such a mound of health issues. I knew of a couple of things, that can go wrong with a weak system, but I wasn't aware of cancer being number one on the list. I'll tell you one thing, my Aloe Life Juice, and Cand Elim went directly to the core, loosening up that fungus, flushing it out! All that we eat, and drink needs to exit our bodies, regularly. Two – three bowel movements, per day is the norm. Anything less than that, should cause concern. But not to alarm you, it can be reversed by what you consume regularly. When the digestive system is off balance, we may begin to feel sick or sluggish, and of course eating unhealthy will contribute.

With my Aloe Life juice, fresh kiwi, watercress, and blueberries, I can't go wrong, finally my energy has returned! After chemo, and radiation treatments, my skin was dry and brittle, and the same with my hair. The new growth of my hair was still just as displeasing as a scouring pad... a worn out one, to make matters worst. So I began entering searches on the internet, for everything organic. Whenever I'd find one product, it led me to another, then another, then some more. That's when I decided to keep track of all the new natural food, hair, and skin care products that I'd began using, and voila! Here it is folks, all of the organic energy that I managed to macramé into my new life style, has been a long time coming! I'm more than happy, and pleased to hip you to what I've learned, through my past breast cancer experience. Mostly everything used in my house now, is organic. From certain cleaning products, food, and yes... even clothing!

My eyes bulged when I came across www.faer-iesdance.com , which is a website that sells organic clothing folks! I hadn't heard of it, until my search. There are other clothing businesses that carry organic wear, but faeries dance was one I thought I should mention. Their site displays everything from organic gowns and dresses, to undergarments. What I love about them most, is how they give to a worthy cause, and are paying it forward! So please, check out this eco-friendly clothing site, when you have a moment. I'm reminded of how very sensitive, my babies' skin was when they were born. My son had the most sensitive skin as a baby. Until this day he has to wear everything cotton, to avoid breaking out in hives or a rash.

Which used to keep me in and out of my pediatricians office constantly. He even had to drink a specialized formula as a baby, after I had tried numerous others that made him sick. I remember those nightmares. He was a good baby, never crying, always smiling and sleeping though. I loved it, but he made up for it in other ways, with often trips to the doctors'. Thank heavens those days are over! And years ago organic foods, let alone clothing, weren't sold in markets that we usually frequented. They are now, and people are catching on! Honestly, who wants to continuously make visits to a hospital, when they can possibly remedy, certain health issues themselves?

Don't get me wrong, sometimes having your doctors' input is unavoidable. I found this section of this chapter a little more fun, then that of the healthier eating, for the simple fact that I just love FASHION! In the beginning of experiencing chemo, I felt and looked like the ugliest creature you'd ever lay eyes on.

It took some time in developing a healthier self esteem, and hurdling over self doubt. After tiring of all of those beautiful sexy wigs of mine, and revealing who I really was, I loved it! But with much help it would still take a while longer to arrive at total assurance, what helped me along was when I found www.morroccomethod.com. This particular site offers all kinds of natural skin/hair care products, that will have you thinking, "why haven't I tried this sooner?" this is how I react once I happen upon, any website that I believe can be of some help, to anyone. Especially to those of you who may be in search of something new, in replacing years of damage, from chemical exposure.

If your looking for natural scalp repair, browse Morrocco Methods' site, and I bet you'll find more than what you expect. I was at my wits end when I read through, and began using this companies' products. They have something for almost anything you can think of. From natural shampoos, conditioners, organic hair coloring, organic detoxifying products, and natural body soaps, such as seaweed hand made soap, that has a gentle skin toner. Their Chamomile-Aloe Vera hand made soap, is another natural skin cleanser. What I found most interesting about Morrocco Method, is how transcendent they are in leaving no room, for guessing games. You can click on the icon near the product of interest, and read all of the ingredients that it holds.

There aren't any secrets, or hidden messages here,

what you see, is what you see. They sell products for all hair types, no one is exempt, isn't that a major plus! A one stop shop, where you can find all things natural for you, and your hubby too! Yes, the men can use a little smoothing of their rough edges, from time to time. Morrocco Method has been around for over 40 years. It's system thrives off of the belief that offering the finest holistic, hair, and skin care products for women, and men are first priority. They have also been paying it forward with other various organizations, that are standing for a worthy cause. So when I order organic products from them, it's being recycled back into helping someone. That my friend is what it's all about, and I'm tickled pink to present to you, healthful information that you may, or may not have, ever dreamed of! Once happening across www.black-girllonghair.com, it brought to recollection, those days of over processing my hair. And the loathsome feel of that old wretched straightening comb, and a perm, I despised both! But had to do something, because wearing a wig began to look like, I had on a big ole cowgirl hat or something. There was no time in braiding my hair, to fit a wig snuggly over top. So I'd just throw it on, and rush out to work. Boy I couldn't wait, until my hair began growing after chemo was over! It took almost two years, in getting back to a full head of hair. Once it was long enough, what'd I do? Regressed to using perms, which didn't last but only six weeks. What'd I do, like a dummy? Perm it yet again. After attempting to get back into the same old routine, all that hair began falling out. Oh sure, it was lovely… at first, but after the third round, my hair was pitiful. On black girl with long hair's site, I was reintroduced to a better way in taking care of my hair. By finding numerous natural styles, of women wearing their hair, as long or short as they felt comfortable with. And that's the whole thing right there, finding confidence in who you are. I saw natural, yet beautiful fashionable hair styles, and without the adding of harmful chemicals. There were women on the site, modeling naturalism at it's best, and with pride.

I also read extremely healthful tips on the upkeep of natural hair. Which confirms good health starting from the inside, working it's way outwardly. I would say going natural, is up there on a scale with child birth, in my opinion though, I can't speak for anyone else. For me going natural was truly difficult. My two daughters' are also wearing their locks chemical free. Although my older girl takes care of her own hair, I'm relieved in knowing she's kept it natural. That's kind of why I compared the upkeep of natural hair to child birth, because honestly, I didn't know exactly what to do with it. All I knew to do was use perms, or result to the occasional painstaking hot comb. I was so blessed to find this particular site though, because I garnered more confidence in myself, as an African American woman. No longer ashamed of my kinky tresses, or even wearing a weave. I'll wear a weave in a minute honey! This way, the color is there, if that's where I'm headed. Or the length is there if I'd like for it to be, no hassle. And I do my own, which becomes a win, win! As opposed to drowning my scalp with chemicals, but now I know how to maintain, and It's not likely that I'll ever go back to using chemicals in my hair.

The scalp needs a rest, just as well as your overall physical being. But I will never say never, guess I will have to see how it goes. It's been going good, for the past four years, which is a stretch coming from me. www.greenpeople.org is a website, that will have your head spinning folks! On this site I found everything, and I mean everything! You name it, it was there! They even list eco-friendly products in caring for your pets... good stuff. First off, have you ever heard of eco friendly appliances? Well maybe you have, but I hadn't until scanning through green peoples' site. How about, natural home and garden, and organic restaurant listings? That's what I said, "organic res-taurant listings?" Personally, I couldn't believe all of what I had found, through this one site alone. And the information with their green listings of international restaurants was crazy! On green people's web, you can find healthy natural ways in which to enjoy food during your travels

So you'll have an easy time of it, and will feel like your at home. Without having to struggle finding what your used to eating. Well... it won't be the ex-act same, but you'll come pretty close, or even better.

Don't know about you, but I'd rather enjoy someone else's hands to the pots, as opposed to me doing it. After all, that's what vacationing is all about, spoil me honey! Who really cooks while on vacation anyways? Especially if your traveling on business, isn't it great to know you'll find eateries, with wholesome goodness in mind? You'll see what I mean, after searching their listings of organic restaurants, from here to Europe, A-Z. They offer wonderful nutritional counseling services information. They also have detailed information on natural beauty products, and a much needed amount of other organic items. Each website that I've had the pleasure of mentioning will leave you well informed. They're filled with all types of ADVICE. Should you have any questions, their customer service information will be, available to you on most sites. They're not all confined to one or two suggestions for health remedies or an ailment, and that's a plus. Another super food, that will help flush unwanted toxins, is wheatgrass. This particular super food, has been known to shrank tumors, by metabolizing the bodies' enzymes, thus creating a dissolving effect. Every nook, and cranny can be revived through wheatgrass alone. Really any food, that oxygenates cancer cells, is a super food from what I've found. And cancer cannot survive if exposed to oxygen. By eating properly, years of toxicity can be extracted from your bloodstream, from those vital organs, and you will look and feel brand new! You can even purchase wheatgrass seeds, to harvest your own. Herbal teas are also great detoxifiers. Green tea, is number one on that list, it's powerful yet gentle on the digestive system. Flaxseed oil with plain yogurt, is another way to detoxify cancer out. You may add fresh blueberries, almonds, and any other berry that is rich in antioxidants. Unsalted almonds, are extremely high in antioxidants, something I recently learned of. Really you can go ahead, and add anything you'd prefer, try and make sure it's rich in antioxidants though. The first time I made my health drink, I opened the fridge and was tempted to add the much desired undesirables.

I could just taste it, my mouth was watering! What's it going to hurt? Blueberries, cookies, and almonds sounds delightful huh? But... definitely not good for anyone. As much as I loved sugar, cancer craves it more, while destroying healthy cells. So... if you can vanquish temptation you'll be on your way. While writing my memoir, instead of snacking on cookies and chips, I drink plenty of water. Or I may whip up a salad, loaded with fresh berries over spinach leaves, and a delicious balsamic vinaigrette, yummy! Sometimes I sprinkle dried cranberries over my salad, trust me it's delicious. How about meats? Well... I'm no vegetarian, I can tell you that now, but for the past six years I've been ordering organic poultry. Just recently I had spoken at an event where a handful of guests were aware of different foods, and natural supplements that may combat cancer. The majority were not, and this didn't surprise me one bit. Skepticism plays a big role in deciphering whether to trust something new or not. To be honest, I was quite skeptical myself after hearing of a variety of natural cancer killers. However, in order to see wanted results through an alkaline diet, one must be consistent. Think about it, is your health something you turn on and off like a faucet? Certainly not, but an alkaline diet, will help to diminish those tough, cancer cells. So it has to be an everyday thing, and in most cases a diet high in antioxidants, should be practiced like second nature. Because I've heard of horror stories, of people going back to their old diet plan which is not a great idea.

That's when the cancer, can come back with a vengeance, if your doing well don't drop the ball. The longer a person maintains a healthy way of eating, the further along they may be, from receiving an unwanted diagnosis. For a person, who's never been diagnosed with cancer, yet has a diet filled with antioxidants may never get cancer. For some, cancer hasn't intruded upon them, as it has others, and why is that? You ever wonder why though? How does cancer plague one person, and totally by pass someone else? I believe that occurs for a number of reasons. I'm pretty sure by what that lucky person is eating, and how often they exercise, and the big one… the amount of sleep plays a major role, in how their immune system wars against contracting illness. And were you aware of the availability, of an energy neutralizer for your cell phone, computer, television, and microwave oven? An energy neutralizer, is used to protect your body against, harmful radiation coming from our toys. Most everyone I know has a television, uses a cell phone, computer, and other devices for business, or entertainment.

Unfortunately, it's become a way of life. In your spare time, please visit www.healthminutevitamin-creek.com. Here you will find, all of the information you need to know, on an energy neutralizer. If you may have questions, simply call 1-888-747-0726 because they have too many facts, that I'm certain a scientist would be able to decipher with ease, so don't take my word for it, browse to see for yourself. I'm telling you… after carefully scanning this website, you may want to take me on a cruise to Italy, I don't know. Maybe have me over for tea, or take me on a trip around the world… yes?! I'm just saying… you may want to do something to celebrate. I got it, send me an e-mail letting me know how your enjoying the new you. Hopefully you've garnered something from hearing about, adding years to your life, and I'd be so very happy in celebrating with you. www.healthy-recipes.com has the know how in putting the wheels of good health, in motion for you. Here you will find all types of wholesome recipes, amongst other ideas and suggestions, which may have similarities as the aforementioned sites, but be sure to spy out those differences, that's where you'll come out a winner! By taking bits and pieces from each site, leaving clarity on what the combining effects will bring. Possibly a handsome hunk with swagger, or a dazzling diva who's aging gracefully.

More food for thought, as well as… facials? Yes of course, this website takes enjoying cooking, and skincare to a whole new dimension. Various forms are presented on how to peel years of smiles and frowns, away. After smoothing on one of their delicious recipes, as a facial, you'll get the idea. I for one have tried the honey facial, and found that the raw brand works best for me. And it does leave your skin with the feel of firmness, and cotton simultaneously. At least that's what I took from my raw honeyed facial. Some of you may have familiarized yourself, with these pampering practices, but have you ever had an opportunity in basking in an herbal body wrap? Neither have I… but intend on checking that off my to do list. Just as soon as I find the nearest locale, I'm there! On the site it looks so relaxing, like a full bodied pedicure, am I silly or what! Honestly, that's what the herbal wrap looks like. Just sheer spoiling of one's self, and why the heck not, right?! Come on, you can't possibly tell me your exhausted temple, doesn't deserve one of those?! Because you know you do! And you know just who'll foot the bill, that's right, hubby! Ladies come on, make him work for the fruit of your garden, make him pay it forward, huh?! On the other hand, if your independently solo, then good for you, either way it works. Treat your own worthy self to a day spa, of your choosing. Okay back to memoir, y'all know sometimes… I can't help myself. And if it seems, I'm bringing to your attention, something of which you've already known, that's because I… did not know anything about an herbal wrap. And wanted to share that with you. Now if someone mentioned chicken wrap, or burrito wrap that'd be right up my alley. Because I know food, that's my thing. Nonetheless, I've never heard of a natural full body wrap. So please treat yourself to paying a visit to that site, you won't regret the road to self reinvention, it'll place you on.

Now this is something that we all must certainly do, in keeping the largest organ squeaky clean. No matter your height, or how much you weigh, what you look, or smell like, we all need this, that's right for our bodies! Are you aware of the fact that, hot showers may cause cancer? Through my own factual research, I've learned of how CHLORINE absorbs into the open pores. When that occurs, the chlorine enters the bloodstream, increasing exposure to toxins. Which may cause cancer, but it's not an over night type of thing, it comes from repetition. Here's how to remedy this dilemma, simply install a filtered shower head, just as you would for your, faucet or drinking water. Most of you may have had one in place, and that's great! Really, it's that elementary, go figure? And it makes sense, for something you'd guard your insides against, why not use that exact mechanism on the outside of the body? I compared this to a similar scenario, like when a person has too much sun exposure. Over a period of time, they may develop skin cancer. But if not enough of your skin is basking in the sun for at least 15 minutes per day, then your level of vitamin D may become deficient. Which can very well mean your lacking the normal in take of vitamin D in your food, or drink. When all along what's needed is a balanced amount of certain nutrients, along with a moderate span of time spent doing outdoor activities.

So it's a mess if you do, a mess if you don't, where lies the middle ground? I'll tell you… it reverts back to us, on how to keep abreast on matters that concern overall health. Seems like the more time progresses, the more we'll need in staying healthy. Believe it or not, some of the most dangerous toxins, are still right under our noses. We've been using them for years, keeping them stored around our homes, in our garages, and under our bathroom and kitchen sinks. What I do now is read labels, for EVERYTHING. Go ahead… leave it to me, and we'll all be out in the woods, sitting around a campfire singing Kumbya! Getting back to nature, who's with me?!

Can you imagine… what life must have been like, way back in the day? I'm talking a couple hundred, or several hundred years. When there weren't cell phones, computers, or cars. The ozone layer was complete, and there was no such thing as processed food.

People were nature savvy back then, they weren't concerned with longevity it was a given, and folks had more consideration for nature. One thing for sure, the earlier generations were up against some pretty nasty diseases. But with having less of a burden, of dealing with less exposure than we do now of other issues. I for one, would not have wanted to live hundreds of years ago, due to other things that were going on, during that era. I certainly would've loved the simplicity though, and naturalism in which they lived.

I had to do an inventory, of cancer causing agents that I'd been using. Some were house hold cleaning products, and there were a couple more personal items, like deodorant, and other cosmetics. Certainly not everything will cause cancer, however... there's a long list that will. Honestly... the more I research, the more I find. We all just need to keep an eye out on what we consume. Developing an exercise routine, also helps relieve stress, and will keep the body functioning, at an optimal level. I used to ignore articles, that talked about eating healthier and exercising. Guess what though? I'm a believer, and a receiver now! I'am, and as a result of doing those things I feel, look, and smell better too. Without clogging my pores with over chemically based deodorants, and perfumes. The all natural woman that I'm now seeing in the mirror, has come a very long way, with still more to go. I had to mesh exercising and eating right into my routine, it was no easy feat, but it became a priority at the top of my list. And what about those hundreds, of hours of sleep that we lose, and can't ever get back? No use in crying over lost sleep. Try developing a new self-care plan, extending your years creating a healthier you. So get those extra winks in before dashing out, mingling with the hustle and bustle that we just can't stay away from.

Green Thumbs Up!

HEY! REMEMBER THAT feeling you had, on the day you graduated high school? Or when you graduated from college, how'd you feel? Those nights, spent burning the midnight oil studying, weren't for naught, and the end result? Your head held high, gliding across that stage clad in your cap, and gown. Camera lights flashing from proud relatives, or friends seizing your moment! Didn't it feel great to achieve those accomplishments?! But with much sacrifice, and a made-up mind... you had a goal, a vision. You saw yourself sitting in that auditorium, listening to your professor presenting his lecture. You walked that University campus, in your mind long before move-in day. That's what it's all about, dreaming, visualizing, planning, and doing. All of your many dreams would have been just that. Instead... your motivation, forged the initiative toward perseverance, and optimism landed you in the winners circle. I'm certain that it wasn't all peaches and cream. So congratulations, my hats off to you, and as a bonus you get two green thumbs-up!

My experience with cancer was out of this world, straight to the moon! But ultimately… I had gained, more than what was lost. By not giving in nor giving up, and keeping it moving. We may not always realize, the strength that lies within until faced, with a challenge. I acquired self-confidence, and met challenges with determination. I had to survive… not as a defeated single-parent, but as the strong woman I was born to be! I had to make an example for my children by setting a standard, showing them and by going through the motions. Right before their eyes, they witnessed raw survival. They saw me never complaining, and overwhelming anyone with my responsibilities, and burdens of my circumstances. I hadn't even mentioned having breast cancer, to my children in the beginning.

Eventually I had to, but at the time I felt bad about keeping them in the dark. I didn't expect my two younger children to understand that at all. But my oldest was 10 years old, and could grasp my life-threatening secret. Once She noticed my hair falling out, that's when I had some explaining to do. I answered her questions, and reassured her that I'd be okay. She cried and cried, and my talking to try and ease her mind didn't help, so I just showed her that mommy would be alright by facilitating a continual safety net. My children saw me as their security blanket, and naturally parents should be. It took hard work, in not allowing the circumstances to capsize our unit.

Even being homeless, didn't affect us as I had perceived it would. The most I would say, my children had an issue with, was moving away from their old friends, and that was difficult in and of it self. There were days when they'd give me a hard way to go, because we had moved to the shelter. Sometimes my eldest would treat me as if the roles were reversed, I was the child, she was the adult. When she'd voice her opinion of how she felt about anything, most of the time I'd listen, as a child. Fair enough... as adults don't we need to vent at times? So do children, they need to get frustrations out, but in a certain manner. Okay I gave her that, along with just enough rope. Because there were moments, not too often but there were instances where I had to remind her, of how her bread was being buttered, and who was providing the milk honey. My daughter at ten years old was very bright, and that's how I approached her. So when she got too big for her bridges I had to remind her, that she had a loving father. And he'd be willing for her to live with him, if we had to come to that fork in the road.

I made it clear that I could not help the circumstances at the time, but they would get better. She understood that it would happen, whether she stayed with mama or not. I wasn't at all setting out to be mean or hurt her feelings, I was being honest. After all... her dad lived in the neighborhood that we moved away from, in close proximity of all her friends, it was a sweet deal. What more could she possibly have wanted? I gave her space to think about it, and had even taken it a step further in discussing it with her dad. He hit the ceiling because he wasn't ready, and still isn't even though she's with him now. But she is almost eighteen so really, a portion of the tough part has past, but only a teaser of a portion. And that's all I'll say about that.

My cancer experience, in its entirety taught my children, and I a great deal though. I learned how to take better care of myself, and as young as my children were at that time they were watching. My son, and eldest daughter remember the struggle, and how we overcame. They were able to partake of a life-changing milestone, and we reached it together. I saw to it that our bond would outlast the storms, and it has. Even though my eldest now lives with her dad, what she took with her, will keep her grounded. Recently she professed of how she wishes we were close like we used to be. She regrets some things that caused me to move her to her dad's house.

Unbeknownst to her, during that phone call, I was bawling my eyes out. We as parents don't always have the answers that our children need, but we have that intuition and knowing what's best for them. So I give my girl two green thumbs-up as well! It lets me know, that in light of what had happened to cause those circumstances, she was paying attention. Our conversation was mainly about forgiveness, something she had learned from me over the years. And I'm so glad I taught her that, in order to be forgiven you must forgive. I was asked what was the highlight of the breast cancer experience? The pivotal moment as mentioned earlier, was when I saw an off-duty nurse waiting for her chemo treatment. Either she was coming from, or going to work.

That's when I concluded that I could do it. One biweekly treatment at a time. It was a gradual process, that I didn't whip up instantaneously, but I had to pick up the pace. I faced the music, and removed my running shoes. I was so used to running away from everything, but not this time. To save my own life, and continue fighting I had to stop running! And then I was asked, what type of advice would I give to someone recently diagnosed? Are you sitting? It may take a few minutes. Seriously though, I would advise you, to do you! That's right!

Disengage yourself from anything that causes you stress. Make people understand, the importance of your peace of mind. Re-prioritize your life, what's more important than your longevity? Develop a healthy diet, and this can also be uncertain, because fresh fruits and veggies contain bacteria's, that can be detrimental to someone, receiving chemotherapy. Some vitamins pose a risk as well, but I will say this, discuss, discuss, and discuss, everything with your doctor. I was told to only eat canned fruits and vegetables. After the fact, I had learned of the many alternatives to Chemo through my own research.

Being that everyone's DNA is unique, it's best to err on the side of caution. How about a makeover? Whether you've had, or have hair loss you don't have to appear as a cancer patient. When I underwent cancer treatment, I wore a different color wig or scarf every day. They were just accumulating out of control, and I began to love it! I had beautiful burgundy, brilliant blonde, cutie patootie brown, and lovely purple lavender. They were top-quality gorgeous wigs, and also lifted my spirits during those blue moments. On the final day of Chemo Therapy, and the last surgical procedure I had graduated! Almost seven years later here I am, sharing my survival story! Something else you may find helpful, is joining a local support group. You will be encouraged, by getting involved, and listening to other people's experiences. You'd be surprised, at what you could take away from it.

As essential as it was, I never had time to join a support group, but wished I would've. Nevertheless, I had joined a church and had met people along the way, who in turn became a strong support network. Having to work two jobs, during chemo didn't allow much time for anything. But... I managed a transition from a worry wart, into a confident cement strong breast cancer survivor.

And my garden is now plenteous in love, and

patience. With a good measure of nourishment, it has blossomed into a splendor for the eyes to behold. Needless to say, we've all gone through stormy seasons haven't we? When the tough times arise just know, trouble doesn't last always. When your tomorrow turns into today welcome it. A new place in time, you've never seen before. Yesterday is but a memory, not forgotten but cherished and true. I now look over the horizon, with a brilliant light looming over my garden, it's beautiful. I've found merriment, while basking in its resilience. If it hadn't been for the down pouring of storms, my God! I wouldn't had recognized the sun shining. Always remember to love some one each day, as loving yourself. May God richly bless you all. I won't say THE END, but will say…

…THE BEGINNING!!

Final Thoughts

MORE THAN YOU'LL ever know I'am so grateful to you, in allowing me—another human being, an opportunity in sharing this intimate space. Words can not explain my gratitude, and my prayer on this day? Is for you to be, and feel the energy of blessed assurance. Till I Grow, will hopefully have reached a part of you, once encompassed or tarnished with pain, loss, regrets, and anything else that may have taken you out of your comfort zone. To be presented with an unexpected experience, where you thought you were trooping alone. Thank God I'm here to tell you, your never alone. Always remember to take time and smell the roses! For as pleasing as a garden is to the eyes, it's more inspiring to know, that it lives and breaths without a care in the world, and God tends it with His everlasting provisions, as He will you. Stand tall and keep it moving, may God bless you forever and a day!